Psychosocial Impact of Lupus
Social Work's Role and Function

Edited by
N. L. Beckerman and Charles Auerbach

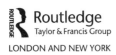

Routledge
Taylor & Francis Group

LONDON AND NEW YORK

First published 2013
by Routledge
2 Park Square, Milton Park, Abingdon, Oxon, OX14 4RN

Simultaneously published in the USA and Canada
by Routledge
711 Third Avenue, New York, NY 10017

Routledge is an imprint of the Taylor & Francis Group, an informa business

British Library Cataloguing in Publication Data
A catalogue record for this book is available from the British Library

ISBN13: 978-0-415-81651-9

Typeset in Garamond
by Taylor & Francis Books

Publisher's Note
The publisher would like to make readers aware that the chapters in this book may be referred to as articles as they are identical to the articles published in the special issue. The publisher accepts responsibility for any inconsistencies that may have arisen in the course of preparing this volume for print.

Contents

Citation Information

The following chapters were originally published in the journal *Social Work in Health Care*, volume 51, issue 7 (2012). When citing this material, please use the original page numbering for each article, as follows:

Preface
Originally published with the title: "Introduction to the Special Issue: Psychosocial Impact of Lupus: Social Work's Role and Function"
N. L. Beckerman and Charles Auerbach
Social Work in Health Care, volume 51, issue 7 (2012) pp. 573-575

Chapter 1
Systemic Lupus Erythematosus: An Overview
Anca Askanase, Katrina Shum and Hal Mitnick
Social Work in Health Care, volume 51, issue 7 (2012) pp. 576-586

Chapter 2
SLE: Serving the Underserved in an Academic Medical Center
Irene Blanco
Social Work in Health Care, volume 51, issue 7 (2012) pp. 587-596

Chapter 4
Listening to Lupus Patients and Families: Fine Tuning the Assessment
N. L. Beckerman and Michele Sarracco
Social Work in Health Care, volume 51, issue 7 (2012) pp. 597-612

Chapter 5
Locus of Control and Lupus: Patients' Beliefs, Perspectives, and Disease Activity
Charles Auerbach and N. L. Beckerman
Social Work in Health Care, volume 51, issue 7 (2012) pp. 613-626

Chapter 6
Lupus and Community-Based Social Work
Wendy Schudrich, Diane Gross and Jessica Rowshandel
Social Work in Health Care, volume 51, issue 7 (2012) pp. 627-639

Chapter 7

Patients With Lupus: An Overview of Culturally Competent Practice
Carmen Ortiz Hendricks
Social Work in Health Care, volume 51, issue 7 (2012) pp. 640-651

Chapter 8

Research Studies and Their Implications for Social Work Practice in a Multidisciplinary Center for Lupus Care
Su Jin Kim, Pretima Persad, Doruk Erkan, Kyriakos Kirou, Roberta Horton and Jane E. Salmon
Social Work in Health Care, volume 51, issue 7 (2012) pp. 652-660

Preface

N. L. Beckerman and Charles Auerbach

This book is devoted to enhancing the knowledge and skill of social work practice with patients and families living with systemic lupus erythematosus (often referred to as lupus). SLE is a chronic autoimmune disease with acute periodic flare-ups of symptoms impacting skin and inflammation of joints. One typical symptom is a "butterfly" rash over the cheeks and the bridge of the nose that may resemble the markings on a wolf's face (lupus is Latin for wolf). For some patients, organ involvement can result in life threatening complications (Lupus Foundation of America 2001; Seawell & Danoff-Burg, 2005). It is a chronic illness that may require powerful medications that can have very difficult side effects to tolerate (Moses, Wiggers, & Cockburn, 2005). Lupus is representative of many autoimmune disorders in which one must cope with chronicity, and acuity and medication side effects simultaneously.

Lupus is estimated to affect as many as 1.5 million Americans (Lupus Foundation of America, 2001). Women are more likely than men to have the disorder at a ratio of 9:1, and lupus disproportionately affects women of color (Moses, Wiggers, Nicholas, & Cockburn, 2005). For the majority of patients diagnosed with lupus, there are significant functional and emotional challenges and a high degree of psychological symptoms such as anxiety, depression and mood disorders (Seawell & Danoff-Burg, 2005). Patients are often overwhelmed and uncertain and social work can be a primary source of support across the health care continuum. This book provides an overview of the various components of the social work role and function with those living with lupus.

The opening chapter, written by Dr. Askanase, Dr. H. Mitnick and Katrina Shum from NYU Rheumatology, provides a medical primer, a Lupus 101, so that the rest of the articles can be understood with an informed context regarding the nature of the disease, diagnosis issues, common lupus manifestations, treatments and side effects.

With the medical context provided, Dr. Irene Blanco from Albert Einstein College of Medicine offers a more hands on overview of how lupus presents in her clinics and with her patients. This is an urban population that represents the national epidemiology, almost exclusively women, and largely women of color. She looks at the interplay between the illness and the psychosocial and socioeconomic factors that mutually influence one another. Her article, "Serving the Underserved" serves as an example for other urban settings with Lupus clinics.

Dr. Rosemarie Cartagine, an Integrative medicine practitioner shares a holistic overview of working with those affected by Lupus. In her chapter, "Lupus: An Integrative Medicine perspective to assessment and treatment of an autoimmune disorder", she explains the tenets of Integrative Medicine (IM) and takes a multi-faceted, approach to patient care, integrating traditional medicine with the more natural complementary and alternative medicine modalities. She discusses this healing-oriented approach as it relates to the assessment and treatment of a patient challenged by common yet bedeviling symptoms of Lupus.

Before moving deeper into other professional viewpoints of how Lupus affects the patient and family, we share the perspectives of patients and families living with lupus. Several families shared their experiences, their challenges and advice in their own words. This chapter by Beckerman and Sarracco captures both the unique and common psychosocial challenges for the patient and family member. The authors suggest how sensitivity to these psychosocial challenges can be integrated into assessment and counseling with Lupus patients.

Wendy Schudrich, Diane Gross and Jessica Rowshandel provide an overview of the social work role and function in a large community based organization; the SLE Lupus Foundation of New York. This discussion offers a profile of typical issues their clientele present and lessons learned about providing a range of community based social work programs to this population.

Drs. Auerbach and Beckerman report on a study (n=378) that explained how lupus patients' perceptions and beliefs about their illness can influence their experience of the illness. This is a critical component in assessment because if patients believe they have no control, they find that they are more vulnerable to depression and potentially to disease activity. The patients' perception of their illness is an important area of assessment and intervention for social work to continue to focus on as literature demonstrates cognitive behavioral approaches may be particularly helpful with lupus patients.

As the overwhelming majority of patients are women, and in fact, women of color, social work and other health care providers have a responsibility to review the cultural diversity competencies. Dr. Carmen Ortiz Hendricks, a leading scholar in cultural diversity social work education, shares her expertise in this area as it specifically applies to those living with lupus. NASW cultural competencies are reviewed and demonstrated and a variety of other cultural competency pitfalls, issues and practices are provided.

Finally, there must be ongoing empirical research in this area of social work practice; consequently, the Hospital for Special Surgery (Mary Kirkland Center for Lupus) was invited to participate with a brief report of their numerous areas of psychosocial research. We thank the authors who shared their expertise to expand our understanding of this complex disease. We want to thank the patients and their families who also generously shared their lives and their stories with us, so that we can strive to provide the best and most responsive care to this population. Their resilience and strength is an inspiration.

References

Lupus Foundation of America (2001) Lupus Foundation of America, INC. (2001) Fact Sheet. Lupus Foundation of America

Moses, N. Wiggers, J., Nicholas, C., & Cockburn, J. (2005). Prevalence and correlates of perceived unmet needs of people with systemic Lupus Erythematosus. Patient Education Counseling, 57 (1), 30-38.

Seawell, A., & Danoff-Burg (2005). Body image and sexuality in women with and without Systemic Lupus Erythematosus. Sex Roles, 53, (11-1

Systemic Lupus Erythematosus: An Overview

ANCA ASKANASE, MD, MPH, KATRINA SHUM, BS,
and HAL MITNICK, MD

Department of Rheumatology, NYU School of Medicine, New York, New York, USA

Systemic lupus erythematosus (SLE) is a systemic autoimmune disease of unknown etiology in which the normal immune responses are directed against healthy organs and tissues. The disregulated immune system produces antibodies that attack the skin, joints, kidneys, heart, and brain. Some people experience mild rashes and arthritis, others suffer debilitating fever, fatigue, joint pain, and severe organ and/or life-threatening disease. This article provides a medical overview of the epidemiology of SLE, the challenges of diagnosing SLE, the complexity of the clinical manifestations and treatment issues, and the impact of SLE on patients' lives. We also discuss the progress in understanding the disease and its therapy over the last century.

INTRODUCTION

Systemic lupus erythematosus (SLE) is a systemic disease of unknown etiology in which the normal immune responses are directed against the body's own healthy tissues. Lupus is a disease in which the immune system becomes overactive, producing antibodies that attack various tissue and organs, including the skin, joints, kidneys, heart, and brain. While some people experience only mild rashes and arthritis, others suffer debilitating fever, fatigue, joint pain, or severe organ and/or life-threatening disease (Lahita,

1

2004). For the purposes of this article, the terms SLE and lupus will be used interchangeably and refer to the same systemic illness.

Epidemiology

SLE is a rare disease with an estimated prevalence of 1 per 144 Black females (>18 years old) as opposed to 1 per 492 White females (>18 years old) (Chakravarty, Bush, Manzi, Clarke, & Ward, 2007), consistent with an increase risk in Blacks of African-American descent. It is more common in women. The female to male ratio in adults is approximately 9:1 (Urowitz, et al., 2011). By age, the female:male ratio is 3:1 before puberty, an incredible 10–15:1 during childbearing years, with a slight decrease again after menopause, 8:1 (Lahita, 1999). The peak age of SLE diagnosis is between 15 to 44 years. Though rare, the number of patients with SLE is not trivial. Estimates of patients suffering from SLE in the United States alone range from 300,000 to 4 million people (Lim et al., 2009).

The disease has a strong genetic component and familial aggregation. Familial prevalence was found to be 5.6% if one first degree relative is affected (Alarcon-Segovia et al., 2005). Disease concordance in dizygotic twins is 2–5%, and in monozygotic twins 29–57% (Michel et al., 2001; Moser, Kelly, Lessard, & Harley, 2009) suggesting that while genes are important they are not the only cause. Environmental factors are presumed to play an important role in disease development and incomplete expression in monozygotic twins support this concept.

Diagnosis Issues and Clinical Manifestations

For research purposes and the clinical identification of lupus patients, most rheumatologists agree that the *1982 American College of Rheumatology (ACR) Criteria* for diagnosis of SLE are *very important* (Tan et al., 1982). These were revised in 1997 (Hochberg, 1997). Patients who do not meet criteria, may nevertheless have similar disease manifestations and respond to therapies noted below.

The criteria include a set of clinical and laboratory features which are listed with their respective prevalence in lupus in Table 1. Table 1 also includes other common laboratory markers. The descriptions of each criterion and ACR diagnostic threshold are as follows:

Clinical Criteria

1. The **butterfly rash** is characterized by a facial fixed erythema that can be flat or raised and spares the nasolabial folds.
2. The **discoid rash** are defined as raised patches, adherent keratotic scaling, or follicular plugging anywhere on the body. Older discoid lesions can cause hyper or hypo-pigmented scarring.

TABLE 1 SLE Manifestations

Manifestation	Presence in SLE patients
ACR Clinical Criteria	
Butterfly Rash	80–90%
Discoid Rash	
Photosensitivity	
Oral Ulcers	50–70%
Arthritis	76–100%
Serositis	30%
Renal Disease	50%
Brain Disease	
Seizures	15%
Psychosis (organic mental syndrome)	20%
ACR laboratory criteria	
Hematologic Criteria	
Hemolytic Anemia	5–40%
Leukopenia	60%
Lymphopenia	60–84%
Thrombocytopenia	60%
Immunologic Criteria	
Anti-dsDNA	40–70%
Anti-Smith	15–55%
Anti-Phospholipid	25–50%
Antinuclear Antibodies	
Other laboratory markers, but not part of criteria	
Anemia of Chronic Disease (Hct < 35%)	57–78%
Neutropenia	
Anti-RNP	30–80%
Anti-SSA/Ro	35–60%
Anti-SSB/La	10–15%

3. **Photosensitivity** refers to the skin rashes from sunlight described by the patient history or seen by a physician.
4. **Oral or nasal ulcers** are usually painless and must be observed by a physician.
5. **Arthritis** in lupus is typically non-erosive, non-deforming, and frequently precedes other manifestations of SLE. It is associated with morning stiffness, can be evanescent or persistent, affects the knees and the small joints of hands (PIPs), and produces objective evidence of inflammation (tenderness, swelling, effusion). It may result in reducible deformities referred to as Jaccoud's arthropathy.
6. **Serositis** may present as painful or painless pleural, pericardial, or ascitic fluid collections (i.e., fluid in the chest and abdominal cavities). This indicates inflammation of the lining of lung, heart, and abdominal structures. However, only pleurisy and pericarditis are classified as criteria.
7. **Kidney disease** is defined by persistent hematuria (not criteria), proteinuria, or cellular casts. This is one of the most common organ threatening manifestations of SLE occurring in as many as 50% of patients.

8. **Brain disease** in lupus can be manifested in different ways. However, seizures or psychosis (organic mental syndrome), although rare, are the most characteristic central nervous system (CNS) manifestations of the disease and as such have been included as criteria. Other neurospsychiatric (NP) manifestations in SLE might include common features such as headache, mood disorders, and cognitive dysfunction to rarer events such as seizures, psychosis, and myelopathy. The reported prevalence of NP disease in patients with SLE has varied from 37% to 95% (Hanly, 2008).

Laboratory criteria

9. **Low blood cell counts** (white, red, platelets).
   • Hemolytic Anemia with reticulocytosis.
   • The following low blood cell counts on 2 or more occasions: Leukopenia ($<4,000/mm^3$), Lymphopenia ($<1,500/mm^3$), Thrombocytopenia ($<100,000/mm^3$).
10. **Specific autoantibodies** (anti-DNA, anti-Sm, APL).
   • Anti-DNA: diagnostic marker for SLE and possible renal disease.
   • Anti-Sm: diagnostic maker for SLE and possible CNS disease.
   • Positive finding of APL antibodies, associated with thrombosis, stroke, fetal loss, and thrombocytopenia. The APL antibodies can be recorded as follows:
      • An abnormal serum level of IgG or IgM anticardiolipin (ACL) antibodies,
      • A positive test result for lupus anticoagulant using a standard method, or
      • A false-positive test result for at least 6 months confirmed by *Treponema pallidum* immobilization or fluorescent treponemal antibody absorption test.
   Other antibodies often associated with lupus, not included in the criteria, are as follows:
   • Anti-RNP, also found in mixed connective tissue disease, progressive systemic sclerosis, and arthritis.
   • Anti-SSA/Ro and anti-SSB/La, also found in Sjogren's syndrome with dry eyes and dry mouth, and associated with neonatal lupus.
11. **Positive Antinuclear antibody (ANA).**

A definite diagnosis of lupus requires 4 of 11 criteria present. Other features supporting the diagnosis of SLE include alopecia, fatigue, fever, and Raynaud's syndrome.

Comorbidities: SLE patients develop premature atherosclerosis, their risk of heart attacks and strokes is 10 times higher than that of their age matched controls, and SLE is now considered an independent risk factor for cardiovascular disease (Manzi et al., 1999).

DISEASE COURSE AND TREATMENT ISSUES

Lupus is a disease manifested by "flares"—periods of increased disease activity. Because of the variable nature of this disorder, activity and severity must be assessed repeatedly over time for the presence of new signs or symptoms and/or worsening signs or symptoms in the involved organs. Rheumatologists will also rely on blood tests to predict and verify the presence of such flares. Typically, blood tests will show anti-DsDNA antibodies rise and the complements (C3 and C4) fall with disease activity. The common inflammatory markers (acute phase reactants such as sedimentation rate and the C-reactive protein) may or my not correlate with disease activity. Disease flares are classified as either mild/moderate or severe based on the severity of symptoms. These definitions help guide treatments, which will target the dysregulation of the immune system.

Mild/moderate flares present as rashes, oral ulcers, and/or arthritis. These flares are often confined to skin and joints and at times also associated with fever and fatigue. Treatment options for mild flares (e.g., malar rash, fatigue, and arthralgia) include antimalarials (such as hydroxychloroquine 200–400 mg), non-steroidal anti-inflammatories (NSAIDs), and steroids (often less than 10 mg). For moderate flares (e.g., more severe skin rash, alopecia), antimalarials might be adjusted or prednisone doses greater than 10 mg might be prescribed. Immunosuppressants, such as Methotrexate or Azathioprine, might be added for a "steroid sparing" effect, for those patients who required prednisone greater than 10 mg to control symptoms. Antimalarial adjustment options for moderate flares might include briefly increased hydroxychloroquine to 600 mg, addition of quinacrine 50 mg Monday through Friday, or a switch to chloroquine. While these medications can help reduce symptoms, improve disease manifestations and sometimes induce remission, they can also have significant negative side effects. Steroids, in particular, commonly cause insomnia, osteoporosis, muscle weakness, and much more. Belimumab (Benlysta) a monoclonal antibody directed against a soluble B lymphocyte survival factor has recently been approved for patients in this category.

Severe flares refer to life or organ threatening disease, such as diffuse ulcerating rashes, significant kidney disease, brain disease, very low platelet or red blood cell count, or bleeding into the lungs. For such severe manifestations of lupus, treatment options include continued hydroxychloroquine 400 mg, consideration of pulse steroid (one gram per day IV for three days) followed by or the addition of high dose prednisone 1–2 mg/kg per day. More potent immunosuppressants, like IV cyclophosphamide (Cytoxan), Mycophenolate Mofetil (CellCept), or recently developed biologic therapies like Rituximab (Rituxan) may be added.

MORTALITY

Recent data from a large international cohort of lupus patients suggest that the 20 year survival in SLE is 70%, a major improvement over the 50% 5-year survival observed 30 years ago (Urowitz, Ibanez, & Gladman, 2005). Another recent study showed that the standardized mortality ratio for people with SLE is 2.4, meaning that a person with lupus is 2.4 times more likely to die of any cause than a demographically matched person without lupus, with the most common cause of death being circulatory disease (Bernatsky et al., 2006). Although the death rate among people with lupus has drastically declined in the past decade with the help of better and earlier treatment, there is still a high incidence of death in young women early in their disease course related to the disease itself or treatment for the disease.

A HISTORIC PERSPECTIVE OF SLE OVER THE PAST CENTURY HIGHLIGHTS ADVANCES IN IMMUNOLOGY, GENETICS, AND PHARMACOLOGY

SLE is a disease that has known great progress during the twentieth and twenty-first centuries. Basic science discoveries to understand some of the pathogenesis of disease as well as evolution in treatment options started in the 1850s when lupus symptoms were first described. A summary of these major advances is shown in Table 2.

The term "Lupus Erythemateux" was coined by the Parisian physician Cazenave in the 1850s. He gave the first description of the facial rash and skin ulceration resembling a bite from a wolf, from which some think lupus (Latin for wolf) derives its name. At about that time in Vienna, the dermatologist Ferdinand von Hebra published the first picture of the butterfly-shaped facial rash (Blotzer, 1983; Lahita, 2004; Smith & Cyr, 1988; Talbott, 1993).

Years later, Kaposi suggested that there are two types of lupus erythematosus: the discoid form and the disseminated form. He described

TABLE 2 Major Advances in Lupus

Use of cortisone	1948–49
Nobel Prize for cortisone	1950
LE prep/IF ANA test	1950–60s
Anti-malarials	1951
Mouse models of SLE	1960 onward
ACR criteria for diagnosis	1982
Cyclophosphamide	1986
Mycophenolate Mofetil	1998
Rituximab	2000
Benlysta	2011

the symptoms characterizing the disseminated form as the following: subcutaneous nodules, arthritis with synovial hypertrophy of both small and large joints, lymphadenopathy, fever, weight loss, anemia, and central nervous system involvement (Kaposi, 1872).

It was not until 1903 that lupus was referred to as a systemic disease. Sir William Osler described 20 young women with skin rashes and chest pain resulting from inflammation of the lining of the lung (pleurisy) or heart (pericarditis). These patients also had fatal kidney disease, strokes, and brain involvement, where 18 died within two years from presentation (Olser, 2009). However, because of improved understanding of the spectrum of lupus we currently recognize that many patients with illness are not as severely ill as Osler described.

Blood tests for SLE, including the LE cell described by Hargraves in 1948 and the detection in the late 1950s of anti-nuclear antibodies (ANA) (Friou, 1957; Hargraves, Richmond, & Morton, 1948; Holborow, Weir, & Johnson, 1957), identified patients with less fatal combinations of disease features. Drug therapy improved over this time; the use of antibiotics prevented infections that were a common cause of death in lupus patients and steroids treated the inflammatory manifestations.

Researchers in the 1950s also discovered two other immunologic markers were associated with lupus: the biologic false-positive test for syphilis (Moore & Lutz, 1955) and the immunofluorescent test for antinuclear antibodies (Friou, 1957). Soon after, the recognition of antibodies to DNA (Deicher, Holman, & Kunkel, 1959) and the other extractable nuclear antigens (nuclear ribonucleoprotein (nRNP), Sm, Ro, La, and ACL) proved useful in describing clinical subsets and understanding the etiopathogenesis of lupus. Particular ANAs, namely anti-dsDNA and ACL antibodies, are now known to be instrumental in certain lupus disease features. Anti-dsDNA antibodies are thought to play a significant role in kidney disease and ACL antibodies are known to be responsible for the "sticky blood" that makes lupus patients more likely to suffer blood clots and/or miscarriages.

As more was discovered in the blood tests for lupus, studies were initiated to understand genetic links. The familial occurrence of systemic lupus was first noted by Leonhardt in 1954 and later confirmed in studies by Arnett and Shulman (Arnett & Shulman, 1976). Familial aggregation of lupus, the concordance of lupus in monozygotic twin pairs, and the association of genetic markers with lupus have been repeatedly described over the past 20 years (Hochberg, 1987).

Other key advances in the understanding of lupus include the development of animal models and the recognition of a genetic predisposition to lupus. The first animal model of systemic lupus was the F1 hybrid New Zealand Black/New Zealand White mouse (Bielschowsky, Helyer, & Howie, 1959). Using these murine models, discoveries have been made in understanding the immunopathogenesis of autoantibody formation, mechanisms of immunologic tolerance, the development of glomerulonephritis, the role of sex hormones in modulating the cause of disease, as well as evaluation of new treatments (Lahita, 1999).

The history of lupus is not complete without a review of the development of treatments. The first reported medication used for lupus was reported by Payne in 1894. He described the usefulness of an antimalarial medication called quinine (Payne, 1894). Four years later, the use of salicylates in conjunction with quinine was proven to be further beneficial (Radcliffe-Crocker, 1898). It was not until the middle of the twentieth century that the treatment of SLE was revolutionized by the discovery of the adrenocorticotrophic hormone and cortisone by Kendall and Hench (1952). Today, corticosteroids are still a major component of therapy for the majority of lupus patients. Antimalarials, as discussed previously, are also still extensively used, primarily for patients with skin and joint involvement, but also as background therapy for more severe disease manifestations.

With the understanding that lupus patients had hyperactive immune systems, immunosuppressants were a logical next treatment for those with severe disease. The burgeoning field of organ transplantation allowed a shared model for suppressing immune responses and attendant inflammation. One of the earliest agents used was Azathioprine. Cytoxan, an alkylating agent derived in the 1960s from WWI mustard gas, saved lives by preventing mortality from kidney failure and other severe lupus manifestations. This was confirmed in a now classic study published in 1986 from the NIH. This trial showed that the combination of Cytoxan and prednisone was superior to prednisone alone in the treatment of lupus nephritis (Austin et al., 1986). In the late 1990s, CellCept was introduced as an alternative to Cytoxan for treatment of severe SLE (Ginzler et al., 2005). Originally developed to prevent the transplant rejection, CellCept down regulates the immune system in a relatively non-specific way (Allison & Eugui, 2000) and was found to improve disease activity in severe SLE patients with fewer side effects than Cytoxan (Allison & Eugui, 2000).

The early twenty-first century introduced a new class of drugs to the treatment of SLE, the biologics, medications created through biologic processes, not chemically synthesized. The first, a drug called Rituximab, targets the B-cells that make antibodies (Pescovitz, 2006), and while this is not specifically directed against those making the lupus-specific antibodies, this is a significant advance over the global inhibition of the immune system provided by drugs like Cytoxan and CellCept. Rituximab has been used for years in patients with B-cell lymphomas with relatively few side effects (Plosker & Figgitt, 2003).

The recent approval of Benlysta by the Food and Drug Administration in 2011, to treat lupus is an important milestone in the efforts to treat this debilitating and potentially fatal disease. This is the first drug approved that was specifically developed for SLE, opening the way to even more effective medicines. It works by suppressing the B-lymphocyte stimulator (BLyS) protein, a key mediator of the immune response. Patients with lupus have elevated levels of BLyS, and it is hoped that inhibiting the protein would quiet the disorder. Phase III clinical trials showed Benlysta, in combination with standard therapy, significantly reduced the severity of symptoms and lowered several blood biomarkers of the disease, compared to standard treatment alone (Navarra et al., 2011).

Living with SLE is a big challenge for patients, mainly due to the unpredictable nature of the disease. Where many patients can cope well and have relatively normal and productive lives, others become their disease. Some patients die because the drugs we use are either inefficient or toxic. Others simply lose a battle of faith when unable to cope with the burden of this devastating disease. They cease to be workers, mothers, daughters, and, instead, become absorbed in the vicious cycle of disability, depression, and distress. It is important for any member of an interdisciplinary health care team to be fully aware of how lupus may affect a patient, as well as an appreciation for the interdependence between the biological dimension of the disease and the psychological sequelae of lupus.

REFERENCES

Alarcon-Segovia, D., Alarcon-Riquelme, M.E., Cardiel, M.H., Caeiro, F., Massardo, L., Villa, A.R., & Pons-Estel, B.A. (2005). Familial aggregation of systemic lupus erythematosus, rheumatoid arthritis, and other autoimmune diseases in 1,177 lupus patients from the GLADEL cohort. *Arthritis & Rheumatism*, *52*(4), 1138–1147.

Allison, A.C., & Eugui, E.M. (2000). Mycophenolate mofetil and its mechanisms of action. *Immunopharmacology*, *47*(2–3), 85–118.

Arnett, F.C., & Shulman, L.E. (1976). Studies in familial systemic lupus erythematosus. *Medicine (Baltimore)*, *55*(4), 313–322.

Austin, H.A., 3rd, Klippel, J.H., Balow, J.E., le Riche, N.G., Steinberg, A.D., Plotz, P.H., et al. (1986). Therapy of lupus nephritis. Controlled trial of prednisone and cytotoxic drugs. *New England Journal of Medicine*, *314*(10), 614–619.

Bernatsky, S., Boivin, J.F., Joseph, L., Manzi, S., Ginzler, E., Gladman, D.D., et al. (2006). Mortality in systemic lupus erythematosus. *Arthritis & Rheumatism*, *54*(8), 2550–2557.

Bielschowsky, M., Helyer, B.J., & Howie, J.B. (1959). Spontaneous haemolytic anemia in mice of the NZB/BL strain. *Proceedings of the University of Otago Medical School*, *37*(9).

Blotzer, J.W. (1983). Systemic lupus erythematosus I: Historical aspects. *Maryland State Medical Journal*, *32*(6), 439–441.

Chakravarty, E.F., Bush, T.M., Manzi, S., Clarke, A.E., & Ward, M.M. (2007). Prevalence of adult systemic lupus erythematosus in California and Pennsylvania in 2000: Estimates obtained using hospitalization data. *Arthritis & Rheumatism*, *56*(6), 2092–2094.

Deicher, H.R., Holman, H.R., & Kunkel, H.G. (1959). The precipitin reaction between DNA and a serum factor in systemic lupus erythematosus. *Journal of Experimental Medicine, 109*(1), 97–114.

Friou, G.J. (1957). Clinical application of lupus serum—Nucleoprotein reaction using the fluorescent antibody technique. *Journal of Clinical Investigation, 36*(6), 890–890.

Ginzler, E.M., Dooley, M.A., Aranow, C., Kim, M.Y., Buyon, J., Merrill, J.T., et al. (2005). Mycophenolate mofetil or intravenous cyclophosphamide for lupus nephritis. *New England Journal of Medicine, 353*(21), 2219–2228.

Hanly, J.G. (2008). The neuropsychiatric SLE SLICC inception cohort study. *Lupus, 17*(12), 1059–1063.

Hargraves, M., Richmond, H., & Morton, R. (1948). Presentation of two bone marrow elements: The tart cell and the LE cell. *Proceedings of the Staff Meeting of the Mayo Clinic, 23*, 25.

Hench, P.S. (1952). The reversibility of certain rheumatic and nonrheumatic conditions by the use of cortisone or of the pituitary adrenocotropic hormone. *Annals of Internal Medicine, 36*(1), 1–38.

Hochberg, M.C. (1987). The application of genetic epidemiology to systemic lupus erythematosus. *Journal of Rheumatology, 14*(5), 867–869.

Hochberg, M.C. (1997). Updating the American College of Rheumatology revised criteria for the classification of systemic lupus erythematosus. *Arthritis & Rheumatism, 40*(9), 1725.

Holborow, E.J., Weir, D.M., & Johnson, G.D. (1957). A serum factor in lupus erythematosus with affinity for tissue nuclei. *British Medical Journal, 2*(5047), 732–734.

Kaposi, M. (1872). Neue Beitrage zur Keantiss des lupus erythematosus. *Archives of Dermatology and Syphilology, 4*, 36.

Lahita, R.G. (1999). The role of sex hormones in systemic lupus erythematosus. *Current Opinion in Rheumatology, 11*(5), 352–356.

Lahita, R.G. (2004). *Systemic Lupus Erythematosus* (4th ed.). Amsterdam, Holland and Boston, MA: Elsevier Academic Press.

Lim, S.S., Drenkard, C., McCune, W.J., Helmick, C.G., Gordon, C., Deguire, P., et al. (2009). Population-based lupus registries: Advancing our epidemiologic understanding. *Arthritis & Rheumatism, 61*(10), 1462–1466.

Manzi, S., Selzer, F., Sutton-Tyrrell, K., Fitzgerald, S.G., Rairie, J.E., Tracy, R.P., et al. (1999). Prevalence and risk factors of carotid plaque in women with systemic lupus erythematosus. *Arthritis & Rheumatism, 42*(1), 51–60. doi: 10.1002/1529-0131(199901)42:1<51:AID-ANR7>3.0.CO;2-D.

Michel, M., Johanet, C., Meyer, O., Frances, C., Wittke, F., Michel, C., et al. (2001). Familial lupus erythematosus. Clinical and immunologic features of 125 multiplex families. *Medicine (Baltimore), 80*(3), 153–158.

Moore, J.E., & Lutz, W.B. (1955). The natural history of systemic lupus erythematosus: An approach to its study through chronic biologic false positive reactors. *Journal of Chronic Diseases, 1*(3), 297–316.

Moser, K.L., Kelly, J.A., Lessard, C.J., & Harley, J.B. (2009). Recent insights into the genetic basis of systemic lupus erythematosus. *Genes and immunity, 10*(5), 373–379.

Navarra, S.V., Guzman, R.M., Gallacher, A.E., Hall, S., Levy, R.A., Jimenez, R.E., et al. (2011). Efficacy and safety of belimumab in patients with active systemic lupus erythematosus: A randomised, placebo-controlled, phase 3 trial. *Lancet*, *377*(9767), 721–731.

Olser, W. (2009). On the visceral manifestations of the erythema group of skin diseases [Third Paper.] 1904. *American Journal of the Medical Sciences*, *338*(5), 396–408.

Payne, J. (1894). A post-graduate lecture on lupus erythematosus. *Clinical Journal*, *4*, 223.

Pescovitz, M.D. (2006). Rituximab, an anti-cd20 monoclonal antibody: History and mechanism of action. *American Journal of Transplantation*, *6*(5 Pt 1), 859–866.

Plosker, G.L., & Figgitt, D.P. (2003). Rituximab: A review of its use in non-Hodgkin's lymphoma and chronic lymphocytic leukaemia. *Drugs*, *63*(8), 803–843.

Radcliffe-Crocker, H. (1898). Discussion on lupus erythematosus. *British Journal of Dermatology*, *10*, 375.

Smith, C.D., & Cyr, M. (1988). The history of lupus erythematosus. From Hippocrates to Osler. *Rheumatic Disease Clinics of North America*, *14*(1), 1–14.

Talbott, J. (1993). Historical background of discoid and systemic lupus erythematosus. In D.J. Wallace, B. Hahn, & E.L. Dubois (Eds.) *Lupus erythematosus* (4th ed., pp. 3–11). Philadelphia: Lea & Febiger.

Tan, E.M., Cohen, A.S., Fries, J.F., Masi, A.T., McShane, D.J., Rothfield, N.F., et al. (1982). The 1982 revised criteria for the classification of systemic lupus erythematosus. *Arthritis and Rheumatism*, *25*(11), 1271–1277.

Urowitz, M., Gladman, D., Ibanez, D., Fortin, P., Bae, S., Gordon, C., et al. (2011). Evolution of disease burden over 5 years in a multicentre inception SLE cohort. *Arthritis Care & Research (Hoboken)*.

Urowitz, M., Ibanez, D., & Gladman, D. (2005, November). *Changing Outcomes in SLE Over 35 Years*. Paper presented at the 2005 ACR/ARHP Annual Scientific Meeting, San Diego, CA.

SLE: Serving the Underserved in an Academic Medical Center

IRENE BLANCO, MD, MS

*Division of Rheumatology, Albert Einstein College
of Medicine, Bronx, New York, USA*

*Systemic lupus erythematosus (SLE) is a multisystemic autoimmune
disorder that can cause significant morbidity and mortality. SLE
typically affects women during their childbearing years, and can
disproportionately affect racial and ethnic minorities. Because this
disease afflicts them at the height of their youth, patients often carry
a large psychosocial burden. This is especially the case in groups
that may have to grapple with other issues such as poverty, work
disability, and lack of insurance. In this review we look at these
issues, and how they affect patients at one major academic center
in the Bronx, NY.*

INTRODUCTION

Systemic lupus erythematosus (SLE) is a systemic illness that can potentially
target all organ systems. While some of the manifestations of SLE are mild
and easily treated, several can cause significant morbidity and mortality. SLE
affects predominantly women in their childbearing years and also disproportionately targets racial and ethnic minorities. The fact that these populations
are targeted at the height of their youth and productivity can cause significant
socioeconomic and psychosocial burden.

On behalf of my colleagues and myself, I thank all of our lupus patients for their humor
and strength and all of the staff that helps us care for them.

EPIDEMIOLOGY

Given the remitting and relapsing nature of SLE, calculating incidence and prevalence rates for the disease is difficult. The incidence of SLE is increasing likely due to more awareness of the condition on the part of practitioners, as well as better diagnostic tests. The overall incidence (per 100,000) of SLE in the United States is currently estimated to be between 0.7–5.0. This number varies significantly in individual segments of the population.

SLE is much more common in women than in men, with a ratio of 9:1. The incidence in women varies from 1.2–11.4, where in African-American populations the incidence rate shoots up to between 3.0–11.0/100,000 (Borchers, Naguwa, Shoenfeld, & Gershwin, 2010; Danchenko, Satia, & Anthony, 2006). Overall there are also higher prevalence rates again in both women and in African-American populations; typically, the prevalence of SLE for African Americans is 2–3-fold higher than for Caucasians (Danchenko et al., 2006). While data is limited about those of Latin-American descent, it appears that incidence and prevalence rates are increased in Hispanics when compared to non-Hispanics (Borchers et al., 2010).

While there are likely environmental factors associated with SLE (such as viral illnesses causing disease exacerbations) as well as hormonal, the disease has a large genetic component. This probably explains why it is found more often in certain populations and families. Although not negligible, the risk of developing SLE in a person with an affected first-degree family member is approximately 8–10%. Often, there are families where multiple members have several different autoimmune diseases (Borchers et al., 2010).

MORBIDITY AND MORTALITY

Despite the fact that SLE is found in all populations, certain groups are more affected than others. Typically, in the United States, African Americans and Hispanics have higher overall SLE disease activity when compared to Caucasians (Alarcon et al., 1998). Not only is SLE more active in these racial and ethnic minorities, but it also tends to be more severe. In the LUpus in MInorities: NAture v Nurture (LUMINA) cohort, African Americans and Hispanics of Mexican descent from Texas were more likely to have renal, cardiac, and hematologic involvement as compared to Caucasians (Alarcon et al., 1999).

Lupus kidney disease can be particularly severe in African-American and Hispanic patients. They not only have higher rates of this SLE manifestation, they are also more likely than other groups to progress to end stage renal disease (Alarcon et al., 2006; Korbet, Schwartz, Evans, & Lewis, 2007). While African Americans also tend to have higher disease damage at presentation, in the LUMINA group, as time went on, it was actually Hispanics that accrued more disease damage. Overall, both African Americans and Hispanics from Texas have higher disease damage than Caucasians (Alarcon, McGwin, Bartolucci, et al., 2001; Alarcon, Roseman, et al., 2004).

While rates have improved since the 1950s, SLE patients continue to have significantly increased mortality. Currently, overall 10-year survival rates are calculated to be between 85% and 95% (Cervera et al., 2003). The cause of death tends to differ depending on the duration of disease. Early on, patients succumb to either their SLE or infections that are brought on from aggressive immunosuppression. However, as the disease progresses, SLE patients have higher rates of morality secondary to cardiovascular disease (Borchers, Keen, Shoenfeld, & Gershwin, 2004). Because of the differences in disease activity between groups it is expected that there are differences in mortality (Cervera et al., 2003). African-American patients have been found to have up to 3-times higher mortality rates when compared to Caucasians (Anderson, Nietert, Kamen, & Gilkeson, 2008; Campbell, Cooper, & Gilkeson, 2008; Kaslow, 1982).

While there are significant differences in morbidity and mortality based on race and ethnicity, socioeconomic factors also contribute significantly to these rates. Multiple studies have shown that income plays a vital role in outcomes in SLE. Poverty and lower levels of education have been found to be associated with a worse physician global Systemic Lupus Activity Measure (SLAM) score (Alarcon, McGwin, et al., 2004). Lower income has also been associated with increased damage accrual and decreased health-related quality of life (Cooper, Treadwell, St Clair, Gilkeson, & Dooley, 2007; Jolly, Mikolaitis, Shakoor, Fogg, & Block, 2010). Patients of lower means have been found to be less adherent with clinic visits. It is unclear though if worse SLE outcomes in those with low income is secondary to non-adherence, access to care or an interaction between race and income (Uribe et al., 2004). Nevertheless, in an analysis of the LUMINA cohort, poverty, not race, was the strongest predictor of mortality (Alarcon, McGwin, Bastian, et al., 2001).

PSYCHOSOCIAL IMPACT

Given the extent of the morbidity and mortality of SLE, it is not surprising that the disease can cause significant psychosocial distress to the patient. Multiple studies have estimated that between 15 and 51% of SLE patients are unemployed or on work disability up to 15 years after the diagnosis. Approximately 40% of patients stop working within 10 years of being diagnosed (Scofield, Reinlib, Alarcon, & Cooper, 2008). Those with lower income levels are two-times as likely to be disabled, while African Americans are actually 7-times more likely to be work disabled from SLE

(Bertoli, Fernandez, Alarcon, Vila, & Reveille, 2007; Utset et al., 2008). The cost of this work disability can be substantial. A 2007 study estimated that the cost of lost wages was actually more than direct medical costs. Several factors associated with these high indirect costs were more disease activity and longer disease duration (Clarke et al., 2008; Panopalis et al., 2007).

Disability and disease activity/damage can cause significant decreases in the quality of life of SLE patients. Multiple validated survey measures, including the Short Form-36 (SF-36) and Health Related Quality of Life (HRQoL) measures have been used to determine physical and mental/social well-being in SLE patients. It has been shown that patients tend to have lower SF-36 scores as compared to healthy individuals (Hanly, 1997). Those with severe manifestations of SLE, such as end stage renal disease from lupus nephritis, have a decreased HRQoL regardless of the degree of their current disease activity. Nevertheless, studies have shown that once disease activity improves, HRQoL improves with it (Fortin et al., 1998; Jolly, 2005). However, HRQoL is not only impacted by disease activity; patients that are unemployed also tend to have lower HRQoL (Bultink, Turkstra, Dijkmans, & Voskuyl, 2008).

African Americans have reported decreased levels of HRQoL from SLE as compared to Caucasians. One study attributed this decrease in quality of life to a sense of disease intrusiveness, where African-American patients significantly felt that SLE interfered with their life to a greater extent than Caucasian or Asian patients (Devins & Edworthy, 2000). Nevertheless SLE patients of all races and ethnicities become frustrated with how SLE affects their lives. Because of the relapsing and remitting nature of lupus, patients often report feelings of uncertainty and anxiety not knowing when another flare will occur (Beckerman, 2011). Often friends and family members do not understand SLE leading patients to feel a sense of isolation (Hale et al., 2006). Like in many debilitating chronic diseases, SLE patients can have difficulty coping with the physical and emotional strain that this illness can take. However, while all patients need help in dealing with their lupus, in one survey of SLE patients, African Americans and Hispanics tended to require more psychosocial assistance than either Caucasian or Asian counterparts (Beckerman, Auerbach, & Blanco, 2011).

Anxiety and isolation, compounded by the financial strains of SLE can lead to feelings of depression (Beckerman, 2011). Disease intrusiveness is also not only related to a decreased HRQoL but also to depression in SLE patients; where disease intrusion often precedes depressive symptoms (Schattner, Shahar, Lerman, & Shakra, 2010). While depression is associated with patient reported disease activity, it may actually have a higher impact on quality of life than SLE activity itself (Carr et al., 2011; Moldovan et al., 2011).

OUR URBAN POPULATION

Our lupus clinics are located in the Bronx, NY. The Bronx is both a county in the state of New York as well as a borough of New York City. It is made up predominantly of racial and ethnic minorities, mostly African Americans (36.5%) and Hispanics (53.5%). It is a young borough—73.5% of the population is under 50 years of age. There is a large immigrant population: 31.4% are foreign-born and 55.1% of all households speak a language other than English at home (www.census.gov).

Many in the Bronx face great hardship. Of all individuals, 28.3% live in poverty as compared to 15.8% in New York State, where it is estimated (as of the 2010 census) that 37.0% of all Bronx families are poor. Of individuals 25 years or older, 30.3% have less than a high school education. This lack of education is of course related to poverty where 46.5% of those people without a high school diploma live below 125% of the poverty level (www.census.gov).

It is safe to assume that this level of poverty in the borough is associated with generally poor overall health outcomes. When we look just at the vicinity around one of our medical centers, Montefiore, three out of every 10 adults rate their health as poor. Our neighborhood is ranked 32 out of 42 New York City neighborhoods with regards to premature deaths. Thirty-three percent of our neighbors have hypertension, one-fourth are obese, and 12% have diabetes. A very large percentage of people in our neighborhood (28%) have no primary care physician, and approximately 30% of our population has been uninsured or lost their insurance over the past year (www.nyc.gov/health). While there are areas of the Bronx with both better and worse health statistics, overall the Bronx fares worse than New York City with regard to health outcomes.

THE EINSTEIN LUPUS COHORT

The Einstein Lupus Cohort (ELC) is a group of patients serially followed in the lupus clinics of two of the teaching hospitals of Albert Einstein College of Medicine, Montefiore and Jacobi Medical Centers. Our cohort is a random selection of our SLE clinic patients that have agreed to be followed for the purposes of conducting clinical research and trials. All patients followed in the cohort have given consent to do so and most of our clinic patients have consented to participate.

Beginning in 2009 we began to collect demographics on our patients to get a better sense of who these patients are and what challenges they may face when confronting their lupus. For the most part our patients are reflective of the Bronx area around them. However, they are not only a reflection of the Bronx but they are also very similar to the SLE patients described in cohorts like LUMINA.

Of the 300 or so SLE patients followed, approximately 57% are African American and 37% are Hispanic. As to be expected of SLE patients, the ratio of women to men in our cohort is 9:1. Approximately half of our patients have a high school education or less and overall about half the patients report making less than $15,000 per year. Given that this is a clinic population and not patients followed in private or faculty practices, most of our patients are on either Medicaid or Medicare.

As in the LUMINA cohort, our patients, who are racial and ethnic minorities as well as from lower socioeconomic strata, carry a significant psychosocial burden as well as an increased burden of disease. A large proportion of our patients have permanent damage from SLE where about 40% have a SLICC Damage Index score of 1 or greater. One-third of our patients have lupus nephritis; many of them have progressed to end stage renal disease requiring dialysis. Several of our patients have had strokes, severe anemias, and life-threatening infections, as well as avascular necrosis of several joints leading to multiple surgeries and joint replacements.

As can be imagined, our patients' extensive disease along with their social issues can pose significant problems for treatment plans and strategies. As in most practices, we have issues with non-adherence to either medications and/or medical appointments. While there is a sub-set of our patients that go against medical advice because of poor judgment, there is also a large group of patients that are non-adherent because of financial constraints, as has been previously been shown in SLE patients (Uribe et al., 2004).

Our clinics meet once a week, during the weekday. Often, when our patients are working, they work in jobs that do not have the benefit of many sick days and vacation days. During a period of illness, despite the fact that they need to be seen often, patients will miss appointments because they are worried or have been explicitly told that they will lose their job because of frequent absences. In these times of economic hardship, this is a risk that our SLE patients are not willing to take, despite the risk of a flare progressing to hospitalization. Also SLE flares can involve many organ systems that require a multidisciplinary team approach. If there are many tests and doctor's visits that cannot be done on the same day, patients may not have a critical study because they cannot take the time from work.

Like the rest of the Bronx, our patients are often in various states of being insured. For a variety of reasons their Medicaid becomes inactive or they are waiting to qualify for Medicare because of their disability. Several have lost their private insurance because of unemployment. This leads to our patients not coming to appointments because they cannot afford to pay for them out of pocket. Waters and colleagues found similar results in California where lack of insurance was associated with fewer physician visits for SLE management (Waters, Chang, Worsdall, & Ramsey-Goldman, 1996). Often because of out-of-pocket expenses from not having insurance, dosages of medications are reduced or stopped all together. For example, a medication like mycophenolate mofetil, that has become essential in the care of lupus nephritis patients, can cost hundreds of dollars per month. To our un-insured patients, even paying for a week or two of medication while waiting for a patient-assistance plan to be instituted can be prohibitive.

Having a stable living environment is a problem for several of our patients. Several patients have lost their housing due to the economy. This has led to quite a few moving in with friends and relatives until new housing can be secured. We have had two patients living in shelters recently, both receiving high doses of immunosuppression. Needless to say, these were less than ideal conditions for patients at such a high risk for infection.

For our patients that have had to move in with family members and friends, it has been a struggle. Most struggle with the loss of independence, and many feel as though they are a burden on their new household. In a recent survey done of our SLE patients, those who live with someone other than their spouse had an increased need for assistance with anxiety (unpublished data). Our adult patients who are cared for by a parent when ill reported needing more assistance with anxiety than those cared for by a spouse (unpublished data).

Unfortunately, this is not the only a source of psychosocial burden. Patients also have difficulty with the socioeconomic burden of living with people that may not be their spouse (unpublished data). A few patients have moved in with friends and relatives that are not much better off financially than they are. This has put even more strain on households that are already stretched thin, leading to a lot of tension and sacrifice on both the part of our patients and their families.

For most of our patients, the histories taken at every visit to our SLE clinics are just as much about their SLE symptoms as about the psychosocial issues that impact their health. While the problems that our patients face can seem insurmountable, being mindful of how a patient's private life impacts his/her health allows for better, more comprehensive care. We have had patients that have become well and gone back to school and work. Others have been able to move out on their own, and take care of themselves and their own families. We have seen our patients through many difficult times, but we have seen them through many happy times as well. We have had weddings, births, graduations, and promotions and being a part of all of these lives has been a privilege and honor.

Of course, we alone have not been solely responsible for our patients' care. Our social workers and patient advocates have been instrumental in helping us and our patients navigate various local, state, and federal agencies. They not only have helped all of us coordinate to get the best care and services possible, but they have served as our patients' counselors and support systems. They have made several overwhelming situations manageable, and without this multidisciplinary approach, we would be at a loss in caring for our patients. Lupus is a complicated disease that is compounded by complicated social lives, acknowledging this only helps us to provide better care through a better understanding of not only out patients' physical determinants of health, but their social ones as well.

REFERENCES

Alarcon, G.S., Friedman, A.W., Straaton, K.V., Moulds, J.M., Lisse, J., Bastian, H.M., . . . Reveille, J.D. (1999). Systemic lupus erythematosus in three ethnic groups: III. A comparison of characteristics early in the natural history of the LUMINA cohort. LUpus in MInority populations: NAture vs. Nurture. *Lupus*, *8*(3), 197–209.

Alarcon, G.S., McGwin, G., Jr., Bartolucci, A.A., Roseman, J., Lisse, J., Fessler, B.J., et al. (2001). Systemic lupus erythematosus in three ethnic groups. IX. Differences in damage accrual. *Arthritis and Rheumatism*, *44*(12), 2797–2806.

Alarcon, G.S., McGwin, G., Jr., Bastian, H.M., Roseman, J., Lisse, J., Fessler, B.J., et al. (2001). Systemic lupus erythematosus in three ethnic groups. VII [correction of VIII]. Predictors of early mortality in the LUMINA cohort. LUMINA Study Group. *Arthritis and Rheumatism*, *45*(2), 191–202. doi: 10.1002/1529-0131(200104)45:2<191::AID-ANR173>3.0.CO;2–2

Alarcon, G.S., McGwin, G., Jr., Petri, M., Ramsey-Goldman, R., Fessler, B.J., Vila, L.M., et al. (2006). Time to renal disease and end-stage renal disease in PROFILE: A multiethnic lupus cohort. *PLoS Med*, *3*(10), e396. doi: 06-PLME-RA-0027R2 [pii]10.1371/journal.pmed.0030396

Alarcon, G.S., McGwin, G., Jr., Sanchez, M.L., Bastian, H.M., Fessler, B.J., Friedman, A.W., et al. (2004). Systemic lupus erythematosus in three ethnic groups. XIV. Poverty, wealth, and their influence on disease activity. *Arthritis and Rheumatism*, *51*(1), 73–77. doi: 10.1002/art.20085

Alarcon, G.S., Roseman, J., Bartolucci, A.A., Friedman, A.W., Moulds, J.M., Goel, N., et al. (1998). Systemic lupus erythematosus in three ethnic groups: II. Features predictive of disease activity early in its course. LUMINA Study Group. Lupus in minority populations, nature versus nurture. *Arthritis and Rheumatism*, *41*(7), 1173–1180. doi: 10.1002/1529-0131(199807)41:7<1173::AID-ART5>3.0.CO;2–A

Alarcon, G.S., Roseman, J.M., McGwin, G., Jr., Uribe, A., Bastian, H.M., Fessler, B.J., et al. (2004). Systemic lupus erythematosus in three ethnic groups. XX. Damage as a predictor of further damage. *Rheumatology*, *43*(2), 202–205. doi: 10.1093/rheumatology/keg481 keg481 [pii]

Anderson, E., Nietert, P.J., Kamen, D.L., & Gilkeson, G.S. (2008). Ethnic disparities among patients with systemic lupus erythematosus in South Carolina. *Journal of Rheumatology*, *35*(5), 819–825. doi: 08/13/0323 [pii]

Beckerman, N.L. (2011). Living with lupus: a qualitative report. *Social Work in Health Care*, *50*(4), 330–343. doi: 936632416 [pii] 10.1080/00981389.2011.554302

Beckerman, N.L., Auerbach, C., & Blanco, I. (2011). Psychosocial dimensions of SLE: implications for the health care team. *Journal of Multidisciplinary Healthcare*, *4*, 63–72. doi: 10.2147/JMDH.S19303 jmdh-4-063 [pii]

Bertoli, A.M., Fernandez, M., Alarcon, G.S., Vila, L.M., & Reveille, J.D. (2007). Systemic lupus erythematosus in a multiethnic US cohort LUMINA (XLI): Factors predictive of self-reported work disability. *Annals of the Rheumatic Diseases*, 66(1), 12–17. doi: ard.2006.055343 [pii] 10.1136/ard.2006.055343

Borchers, A.T., Keen, C.L., Shoenfeld, Y., & Gershwin, M.E. (2004). Surviving the butterfly and the wolf: Mortality trends in systemic lupus erythematosus. *Autoimmunity Reviews*, 3(6), 423–453. doi: 10.1016/j.autrev.2004.04.002 S1568997204000588 [pii]

Borchers, A.T., Naguwa, S.M., Shoenfeld, Y., & Gershwin, M.E. (2010). The geoepidemiology of systemic lupus erythematosus. *Autoimmunity Reviews*, 9(5), A277–287. doi: S1568-9972(09)00217-1 [pii] 10.1016/j.autrev.2009.12.008

Bultink, I.E., Turkstra, F., Dijkmans, B.A., & Voskuyl, A.E. (2008). High prevalence of unemployment in patients with systemic lupus erythematosus: Association with organ damage and health-related quality of life. *Journal of Rheumatology*, 35(6), 1053–1057. doi: 08/13/0321 [pii]

Campbell, R., Jr., Cooper, G.S., & Gilkeson, G.S. (2008). Two aspects of the clinical and humanistic burden of systemic lupus erythematosus: Mortality risk and quality of life early in the course of disease. *Arthritis and Rheumatism*, 59(4), 458–464. doi: 10.1002/art.23539

Carr, F.N., Nicassio, P.M., Ishimori, M. L., Moldovan, I., Katsaros, E., Torralba, K., et al. (2011). Depression predicts self-reported disease activity in systemic lupus erythematosus. *Lupus*, 20(1), 80–84. doi: 0961203310378672 [pii] 10.1177/0961203310378672

Cervera, R., Khamashta, M.A., Font, J., Sebastiani, G.D., Gil, A., Lavilla, P., et al. (2003). Morbidity and mortality in systemic lupus erythematosus during a 10-year period: A comparison of early and late manifestations in a cohort of 1,000 patients. *Medicine*, 82(5), 299–308. doi: 10.1097/01.md.0000091181.93122.55

Clarke, A.E., Panopalis, P., Petri, M., Manzi, S., Isenberg, D.A., Gordon, C., et al. (2008). SLE patients with renal damage incur higher health care costs. *Rheumatology*, 47(3), 329–333. doi: kem373 [pii] 10.1093/rheumatology/kem373

Cooper, G.S., Treadwell, E.L., St Clair, E.W., Gilkeson, G.S., & Dooley, M.A. (2007). Sociodemographic associations with early disease damage in patients with systemic lupus erythematosus. *Arthritis and Rheumatism*, 57(6), 993–999. doi: 10.1002/art.22894

Danchenko, N., Satia, J.A., & Anthony, M.S. (2006). Epidemiology of systemic lupus erythematosus: A comparison of worldwide disease burden. *Lupus*, 15(5), 308–318.

Devins, G.M., & Edworthy, S.M. (2000). Illness intrusiveness explains race-related quality-of-life differences among women with systemic lupus erythematosus. *Lupus*, 9(7), 534–541.

Fortin, P.R., Abrahamowicz, M., Neville, C., du Berger, R., Fraenkel, L., Clarke, A.E., et al. (1998). Impact of disease activity and cumulative damage on the health of lupus patients. *Lupus*, 7(2), 101–107.

Hale, E.D., Treharne, G.J., Lyons, A.C., Norton, Y., Mole, S., Mitton, D.L., et al. (2006). "Joining the dots" for patients with systemic lupus erythematosus: Personal perspectives of health care from a qualitative study. *Annals of the Rheumatic Diseases, 65*(5), 585–589. doi: ard.2005.037077 [pii] 10.1136/ard.2005.037077

Hanly, J.G. (1997). Disease activity, cumulative damage and quality of life in systematic lupus erythematosus: Results of a cross-sectional study. *Lupus, 6*(3), 243–247.

Jolly, M. (2005). How does quality of life of patients with systemic lupus erythematosus compare with that of other common chronic illnesses? *Journal of Rheumatology, 32*(9), 1706–1708. doi: 0315162X-32-1706 [pii]

Jolly, M., Mikolaitis, R.A., Shakoor, N., Fogg, L.F., & Block, J.A. (2010). Education, zip code-based annualized household income, and health outcomes in patients with systemic lupus erythematosus. *Journal of Rheumatology, 37*(6), 1150–1157. doi: jrheum.090862 [pii] 10.3899/jrheum.090862

Kaslow, R.A. (1982). High rate of death caused by systemic lupus erythematosus among U. S. residents of Asian descent. *Arthritis and Rheumatism, 25*(4), 414–418.

Korbet, S.M., Schwartz, M.M., Evans, J., & Lewis, E.J. (2007). Severe lupus nephritis: Racial differences in presentation and outcome. *Journal of the American Society of Nephrology, 18*(1), 244–254. doi: ASN.2006090992 [pii] 10.1681/ASN.2006090992

Moldovan, I., Katsaros, E., Carr, F.N., Cooray, D., Torralba, K., Shinada, S., et al. (2011). The Patient Reported Outcomes in Lupus (PATROL) study: Role of depression in health-related quality of life in a Southern California lupus cohort. *Lupus, 20*(12), 1285–1292. doi: 0961203311412097 [pii] 10.1177/0961203311412097

Panopalis, P., Petri, M., Manzi, S., Isenberg, D.A., Gordon, C., Senecal, J.L., et al. (2007). The systemic lupus erythematosus Tri-Nation study: Cumulative indirect costs. *Arthritis and Rheumatism, 57*(1), 64–70. doi: 10.1002/art.22470

Schattner, E., Shahar, G., Lerman, S., & Shakra, M.A. (2010). Depression in systemic lupus erythematosus: The key role of illness intrusiveness and concealment of symptoms. *Psychiatry, 73*(4), 329–340. doi: 10.1521/psyc.2010.73.4.329 10.1521/psyc.2010.73.4.329 [pii]

Scofield, L., Reinlib, L., Alarcon, G.S., & Cooper, G.S. (2008). Employment and disability issues in systemic lupus erythematosus: A review. *Arthritis and Rheumatism, 59*(10), 1475–1479. doi: 10.1002/art.24113

Uribe, A.G., Ho, K.T., Agee, B., McGwin, G., Jr., Fessler, B.J., Bastian, H.M., et al. (2004). Relationship between adherence to study and clinic visits in systemic lupus erythematosus patients: Data from the LUMINA cohort. *Lupus, 13*(8), 561–568.

Utset, T.O., Chohan, S., Booth, S.A., Laughlin, J.C., Kocherginsky, M., & Schmitz, A. (2008). Correlates of formal work disability in an urban university systemic lupus erythematosus practice. *Journal of Rheumatology, 35*(6), 1046–1052. doi: 08/13/054 [pii]

Waters, T.M., Chang, R.W., Worsdall, E., & Ramsey-Goldman, R. (1996). Ethnicity and access to care in systemic lupus erythematosus. *Arthritis Care and Research, 9*(6), 492–500.

Lupus: An Integrative Medicine Approach to Assessment and Treatment of an Autoimmune Disorder

ROSEMARIE CARTAGINE

INTRODUCTION

Autoimmune diseases are complex conditions. Patients with autoimmune diseases such as Systemic Lupus Erythematosus (SLE) have a plethora of needs that are best served with a multidisciplinary team approach for maximizing the quality of life for patients and their families. This chapter provides an overview of Integrative Medicine as a relevant perspective for assessment and treatment of patients with SLE.

Integrative Medicine (IM) is a relatively new area of healthcare that takes a multi-faceted, whole person approach to patient care, typically integrating traditional medicine with the more natural complementary and alternative medicine modalities. IM is a healing-oriented approach that takes account of the whole person (body, mind, and spirit), including all aspects of lifestyle. It emphasizes the therapeutic relationship between practitioner and patient, and incorporates all appropriate therapies, both conventional and alternative. It is also a fundamentally collaborative approach, which fosters cooperation among the practitioners. The National Center for Complementary and Alternative Medicine at the National Institutes of Health defines IM as "medicine [that] combines mainstream medical and CAM therapies for which there is some high-quality scientific evidence of safety and effectiveness" (The National Center for Complementary and Alternative Medicine).

Integrative Medicine seeks to change the focus in medicine from disease to healing. Sir William Osler (1849 –1919) stated, "It is much more important to know what sort of patient has a disease than what sort of disease a patient has" (Osler). The patient's needs and values inform the course of care while cooperation among clinicians is a priority. Some basic concepts of Integrative Medicine include: the removal of barriers to the body's innate healing response; use of less invasive, natural interventions such as complementary and alternative medicine (CAM) whenever possible prior to or concomitant with more invasive measures; engagement of mind, body, spirit, and community to facilitate healing. In this model healing can always be possible, even when a cure is not (Rakel, 2007). However, chronic illnesses such as SLE require ongoing intervention to manage exacerbations and prevent disease progression. The improvement of the quality of life for persons with SLE can be significantly enhanced through the use of lifestyle medicine.

A pioneering approach to IM was founded by Bland in 1991 when he established the internationally respected Institute for Functional Medicine (IFM). Functional Medicine is a dynamic, patient-centered approach to assess, prevent, and treat complex chronic disease. It addresses the underlying causes of disease, using a systems-oriented approach. This dynamic approach acknowledges that physiological and psychological dysfunctions are the result of lifelong interactions among the environment, lifestyle, and genetic predispositions. The concept is that each patient has unique, complex, and interwoven influences on his or her health status (Institute for Functional Medicine, and Jones, 2006).

In 2011, the Bravewell Collaborative (Horrigan, Lewis, Abrams & Pechura) commissioned a survey of 29 Integrative Medicine centers and programs to determine how IM was being practiced across the United States by (1) describing the patient populations and health conditions most commonly treated, (2) defining the core practices and models of care, (3) ascertaining how services are reimbursed, (4) identifying the values and principles underlying the care, and (5) determining the biggest factors driving successful implementation. The centers included nine of the Bravewell Clinical Network, plus 20 others that met the following parameters: centers directed by either a physician, other doctoral-level healthcare practitioner or nurse; centers in operation for a minimum of three years; patient volume; and/or prior clinical contributions to the field. All the centers in the study were affiliated with a hospital, healthcare system, and/or medical or nursing school. The 29 centers see a total of 19,200 patients per month. The total number of patient visits per month for all centers is about 41,100. The Bravewell findings include: 63% of patients seen were self-referred; the most prescribed therapies in descending order were food/nutrition, supplements, yoga, meditation, TCM/acupuncture, massage, and pharmaceuticals; the four categories of therapies were mind-body, dietary/biological, movement/energy, and manual interventions. The top five clinical conditions for which patients perceive IM to be most successful are, in descending order, chronic pain, gastrointestinal conditions, depression, stress, and cancer. Other conditions treated included but were not limited to: fatigue/sleep disorders, fibromyalgia, immune disorders, and arthritis (Horigan, et al, 2012). Given the findings from this survey, people with SLE can benefit from an Integrative Medicine approach as chronic pain is a common challenge among SLE patients.

The Bravewell study (2011) also reviewed the core values reported by the featured centers. They were asked to rate a series of value statements. The highest rated core values by percentage of influence were: physical (100%), and emotional and mental (97%) influences that affect a person's health are addressed with care that is patient-centered (97%); they teach the connection between lifestyle and health (97%) and encourage patients to take responsibility for their own health (93%), they emphasize CAM modalities (93%), they take into consideration the patient's health goals in the care plan (93%); they address the social influences that affect a person's health (79%) and the care treats the cause of the disease as well as the symptoms (83%). It should be noted that the least important core value listed was the integration of the patient's family and loved ones into the care (41%). This is a significant role a social worker can have in a comprehensive, integrative care plan. Chronic diseases such as SLE can place significant strain on family and friends and, conversely, support from loved ones can have significant positive influence on the quality of life of a person with SLE (Horrigan, et al, 2012).

A patient visiting a Functional Medicine practitioner will likely have a lengthy interview, fill out questionnaires on a variety of topics, and may undergo laboratory tests. The extensive information collected is used to determine the underlying imbalances and influences (whether genetic, environmental, or psychosocial) that have produced the context for disease or dysfunction. The core vectors considered for patients with SLE are nutrition and hydration, stress and resilience, exercise and movement, sleep and relaxation, and relationships and networks/community. Customized interventions are initiated to reestablish balance and functionality, and a comprehensive treatment plan is created to restore health (http://www.functionalmedicine.org/themovement/in-clinical-practice/).

In addition to psychosocial interventions, an individualized lifestyle plan can be developed by social workers and their patients. This would include a comprehensive assessment and subsequent appropriate referrals to practitioners of complementary and alternative medicine (CAM) in the fields of nutrition, acupuncture, herbal medicine, chiropractic, homeopathy, energy medicine, yoga or meditation, with the goal of improved quality of life physically, mentally, socially and spiritually.

An IM approach by definition requires active participation by patients and, ideally, a strong support system to make beneficial lifestyle changes. Beckerman, Auerbach and Blanco (2011) concluded in their study on *Psychosocial dimensions of SLE: implications for the health care team* that "the higher the perceived sense of control over SLE, the less likely respondents were to report feeling depressed and anxious" (p.71). The nature of IM is patient-centered with emphasis on education about the impact of lifestyle on health status, and patient responsibility for his/her own health can give a person living with SLE a greater sense of control possibly leading to a decreased incidence of depression and anxiety.

AN INTEGRATIVE MEDICINE PERSPECTIVE OF SLE

Current theories of the etiology of autoimmune diseases acknowledge not only genetic predisposition to conditions such as SLE, but exposure to an infectious agent whereby the person's immune system becomes dysfunctional or out of balance with an inability to distinguish self from non-self as a probable initiating factor. Integrative Medicine seeks to find and address the underlying cause of disease along with the multitude of factors associated with an autoimmune condition. This includes the assessment of nutritional status, including but not limited to oxidative function, biomere (biological terraine), gastrointestinal integrity, immune system balance (anti-inflammatory) and the hormonal system. Lifestyle interventions include diet, nutrients, stress management, exercise, and emotional and social support.

In his article, Brady (2012) contrasts the allopathic model of treating autoimmune disorders with the use of anti-inflammatory and immunosuppressive agents to provide symptomatic relief to the patient to a more naturopathic or Functional Medicine approach, which seeks to uncover the underlying cause of a condition. He states that "modern research into autoimmune phenomena suggests that radically different approaches may be required [...] including a strong emphasis on very early detection with predictive autoantibodies, a focus on optimizing gastrointestinal mucosal immune function and the microbiome, eradication of infectious agent triggers with antimicrobial therapy" (Brady 2012). He further discusses the coincidence of poor-quality processed foods, which are known to negatively alter the gastrointestinal microbiome (micro-organisms that inhabit the human body with influence on physiology) and often contain a hidden stream of offending dietary antigens, with a higher prevalence of autoimmune diseases. A Functional Medicine approach includes the assessment of a patient's gastrointestinal health as a possible contributory factor in his/her health status. In addition to the presence of parasites or dysbiosis (abnormality of gastrointestinal microflora), intestinal hypermobility may be a contributing factor in the pathogenesis of autoimmune disorders. Nutritional approaches to treatment may include: addressing the issue of leaky gut with effective natural agents, including L-glutamine, N-acetyl-glucosamine, anti-inflammatory botanicals and bioflavonoids, mucilaginous herbs, zinc-carnosine, omega-3-fatty acids, and vitamin D.

Brady summarizes: Physicians should look for immune dysregulatory conditions with a strong emphasis on very early detection with predictive autoantibodies, a focus on optimizing gastrointestinal mucosal immune function and the microbiome, the eradication of infectious triggers with antimicrobial therapy, the detection and elimination of food sensitivities, and the promotion of an anti-inflammatory lifestyle (Brady 2012).

In his review article on CD8+ T-cell deficiency, Epstein-Barr virus infection, vitamin D deficiency, and steps to autoimmunity, Pender postulates that autoimmunity, including SLE, evolves in steps which stem from a deficiency of a component of the immune system, specifically CD8+ T-cell, which is then insufficient to control an Epstein-Barr viral infection. This ultimately ends with immune dysfunction whereby the auto-reactive immune cells (infected auto-reactive B cells) accumulate in a target organ where they produce autoantibodies, thus initiating an autoimmune condition. Pender proposes that, in addition to a genetic deficiency in CD8+ T-cells, a contributory factor in the development of autoimmune diseases is deprivation of sunlight and vitamin D (2012). Therefore, evaluation of vitamin D status can be an integral aspect to management of any autoimmune condition.

A Cochrane review of Dehydroepiandrosterone (DHEA) for systemic lupus erythematosus by Crosbie, Black, McIntyre, Royle, & Thomas (2007) was conducted to assess the effectiveness and safety of DHEA compared to placebo in the treatment of people with systemic lupus erythematosus. DHEA is a naturally occurring inactive steroid, which may possess disease activity modifying properties as well as the ability to reduce flares and steroid requirements. The review concluded that although DHEA demonstrated little or no difference in the disease activity in people with mild to moderate disease, it did improve overall well-being. In people with severe or active disease activity, DHEA may decrease disease activity thereby reducing the need for corticosteroids. Treatment with DHEA was shown to be consistent (to a statistical significance) in the improvement of quality of life of individuals with SLE as opposed to those who had received placebo treatments.

TREATMENT

Natural pain management primarily involves decreasing the chronic inflammation that characterizes chronic pain and immune dysregulation. CAM aimed at dampening pain and inflammation can be used in conjunction with conventional drugs in the early stages of acute treatment. Often natural therapies can be favored as the acute or active phase of the disease diminishes toward a nontoxic approach. Addressing the inflammatory component requires the creation of an anti-inflammatory food plan as dietary practices have a major impact on inflammation. The Standard American Diet (SAD) contributes to increased inflammation through the high intake of saturated fats (found in some cooking oils and fried foods), white sugar and flour, red meat, chemical additives, and dairy products such as milk and cheese. These foods not only increase inflammation but can also invoke allergies, food sensitivities, or immune dysregulation; and interfere with hormone production, cellular integrity, and the function of joints as well as energy production. An anti-inflammatory diet can significantly decrease pain, swelling, and fatigue. A diet rich in whole, unprocessed foods consisting primarily of vegetables, fruits, grains, raw seeds and nuts, beans, and lean protein such as chicken or fish, is nutrient dense. A Mediterranean-style diet incorporates these foods which: provide antioxidants to fight free radicals that damage cells; promote skin and tissue health; repair muscles, tendons, joints and bones; and promote healthy weight and digestion (Kamhi & Zampieron 2006).

Acute care natural therapies may include anti-inflammatory botanicals with analgesic properties such as Salix alba (white willow stem bark), Zingiber officinale (ginger), Curcumin longa (turmeric), or Boswellia serrata (Kamhi & Zampieron 2006). Bromelain, which is found in pineapple, is another well-referenced natural anti-inflammatory. Additionally, anti-inflammatory eicosanoids such as EPA-DHA or alpha-linolenic acid (omega-3 essential fatty acids) are effective in both acute phase and ongoing management of SLE (Kamhi, et al, 2006). Most people are aware of animal sources of the above essential fatty acids, which are found in wild-caught cold water fish such as salmon or sardines. However, due to the concern of toxicity found in fish from such chemicals as PCPs or mercury, it is typically advised to limit consumption of fish to two or three times per week. Therefore it is best to include daily consumption of alternative sources of omega-3 fatty acids such as deep green leafy vegetables, flaxseed and the oil from flaxseed, hemp seed, walnuts and walnut oil, and pumpkin seeds (Kamhi, et al, 2006).

The next phase of treatment for people with autoimmune disorders described by Kamhi, et al (2006) includes the elimination of toxins and support of the natural detoxification mechanisms. Evaluation of digestive function and health including food allergies, intestinal permeability, and colonic microflora (microorganisms in the lower digestive tract) typically is the first stage of a detoxification program. An integrative practitioner may recommend a stool analysis to achieve this. Additional tests may include evaluation of hormone status, especially adrenal and thyroid gland function, oxidative stress profiles, and plasma fatty acids and vitamin D levels.

A patient-centered approach to treatment based on case history, physical examination and laboratory findings would typically include: reducing inflammation, eliminating food sensitivities, and restoring nutrient status and gastrointestinal balance. In addition to nutritional considerations in a treatment plan other CAM therapies may include chiropractic, massage, and oriental bodywork such as acupuncture or acupressure. Physical activity and exercise to improve flexibility, mood, and energy can also be recommended. Emotional support provided by a therapist can be a significant aspect of treatment to afford an individual the opportunity to identify the emotional and/or cognitive influences on his or her health status. Stress reduction techniques such as meditation, prayer, yoga or journal writing are effective self-care tools shown to decrease pain and improve mood. As a patient becomes versed in identifying and minimizing his/her triggers, which may include foods, food preservatives, lack of activity and emotional or mental stress, he/she becomes empowered by a sense of control over his/her health status.

The natural process of inflammation resolution leads to tissue repair and restoration of tissue architecture and function to a normal state. Das (2010) proposes that newer therapeutic strategies to manage lupus and other autoimmune diseases be based on the enhancement of the natural processes of inflammation, wound healing, and repair to diminish side effects. The normal physiology of wound healing can be supported by the inclusion of balanced therapeutic levels of the "healthy fats" such as polyunsaturated fatty acids (PUFAs). A higher ratio of omega-3 to omega-6 fatty acids creates cell membranes that significantly diminish the inflammatory response and provides the structural integrity to cell membranes for healthy tissue repair. Das recommends the inclusion of natural approaches with currently available therapeutic drugs to support the resolution and repair stages of the inflammatory process.

Patavino & Brady (2001) conclude that anti-oxidant and omega-3 fatty acid supplementation has been shown to reduce free radical damage and inflammation, improve immunoregulation, and decrease cardiovascular and renal disease risk. They also state that there may be a benefit to testing for food sensitivities or allergies in order to make beneficial dietary changes that may decrease inflammation.

EXERCISE AND MOVEMENT

A randomized control study to test the efficacy of graded aerobic exercise on fatigue of patients with SLE was conducted by Tench, McCarthy, McCurdie, White & D'Cruz (2003). Ninety-three patients without active disease in any major organ underwent twelve weeks of graded exercise therapy, relaxation therapy, or no intervention. It is commonly known that exercise has been shown to have a positive impact on quality of sleep, depression, fatigue and physical conditioning in healthy individuals. But how would exercise impact patients with SLE? The findings support the use of appropriately prescribed graded aerobic exercise to improve fatigue in patients with SLE. The authors also concluded that there was greater overall improvement in fatigue with the exercise group when compared with the relaxation therapy or no intervention groups. Exercise can be safely prescribed without exacerbating disease activity. Although the study was limited by the small sample size and in the exclusion of patients with very active disease or serious organ involvement, people with mild to moderate SLE can benefit from graded aerobic exercise and ought to be a component of an integrated approach in disease management.

Perandinia, et al (2012) evaluated exercise as a therapeutic tool to counteract inflammation and clinical symptoms in autoimmune rheumatic diseases and concluded that exercise training is a potentially therapeutic tool in counteracting systemic inflammation.

ACUPUNCTURE FOR PAIN RELIEF

Vickers et al, (2012) conducted a systematic review to identify randomized controlled trials (RCTs) of acupuncture for chronic pain in which allocation concealment was determined unambiguously to be adequate. Individual patient data meta-analyses were conducted using data from 29 of 31 eligible RCTs, with a total of 17,922 patients analyzed. Vickers et al concluded that acupuncture is effective for the treatment of chronic pain and is therefore a reasonable referral option. Significant differences between true and sham acupuncture indicate that acupuncture is more than a placebo. However, these differences are relatively modest, suggesting that factors in addition to the specific effects of needling are important contributors to the therapeutic effects of acupuncture.

CASE EXAMPLE

Helena, a 50 year old Hispanic woman, came to our integrative medical offices in 2008. She worked as a Veterinary Hospital Administrator in addition to her dog walking and pet sitting business. She was in a long term, supportive primary relationship and kept pet cats and dogs. Helena reported having been ill since she was 29 years old following an influenza infection, her best friend's and grandmother's deaths, and a love affair that ended. Her health deteriorated over the years and she consulted a variety of specialists who diagnosed her with a number of autoimmune conditions: fibromyalgia, asthma, ankylosing spondylitis, rheumatoid arthritis, multiple sclerosis, and lupus. She underwent many medical treatment protocols including steroid and pain medications, which she discontinued due to limited beneficial results and unwanted side effects. At the time she presented to our offices she was undergoing Remicade infusions every six weeks which exacerbated her fatigue. Due to her concern about long term use of the medications she had been taking and the limited benefit she experienced, Helena decided to pursue a holistic approach for her health incorporating CAM modalities.

When Helena came to our office, she reported that she was frustrated, depressed and discouraged, but not hopeless in her search for solutions to her health issues. Her initial consultation, including history and health survey, revealed many symptoms: muscle and joint pain, migraine, dizziness, extreme fatigue, nausea, sore throat, sinus congestion, breathing difficulties, swollen glands, skin rashes, thyroid nodules, difficulty swallowing, numbness in legs, feet and hands, swollen ankles, heaviness in legs when walking, recurrent low grade fevers, heart flutter, gastrointestinal symptoms of bloating, abdominal cramping, diarrhea, and lesions in her brain, lungs, and pancreas. Helena stated that her most significant stressors were her work and health; prior to treatment in our offices she lost days of work due to her symptoms, especially the extreme fatigue and pain. Her activities of daily living were also severely limited causing further distress.

Upon review of her history she described her childhood as being very stressful. Her father was an alcoholic, her parents separated and she was sent to Puerto Rico where she was primarily raised by her grandmother. She had a few serious injuries in her life including head trauma. She also reported a history of exposure to toxic chemicals, notably numerous pesticides, as well as a recent and historical bout of intestinal parasites. Her surgical history included hysterectomy, tonsillectomy and lumpectomy. Review of her diet revealed that she had a fairly varied diet primarily consuming chicken, turkey or fish, Japanese food, sushi, rice, vegetables, fruit juices, and coffee. She reported being a social drinker consuming about four alcoholic beverages per week. She noted known sensitivity to soy sauce, meat, and gluten, and described her dietary habits as being inconsistent due to the nature of her busy schedule. She also noted that poor eating habits and lack of rest worsened many of her symptoms.

Some of the physical examination findings included severely limited mobility in her joints, palpable tenderness in multiple joints and muscles, positive neurological findings most of which related to poor spinal system function. She was slightly overweight with a waist circumference of 36 inches and body fat percentage of 41.3%. Increased waist size and body fat percentage are associated with a pro-inflammatory state.

Initially care in our offices included gentle chiropractic care, with the addition of massage therapy after a few weeks, followed by nutritional protocols. The goal of care was to improve neural system function, muscular tone, and joint mobility; reduce inflammation; eliminate food sensitivities; and restore nutrient status and gastro-intestinal balance. Her progress was monitored through periodic progress examinations and self-reported evaluation tools such as the Medical Symptoms/Toxicity Questionnaire (MSQ).

The MSQ is a data-collecting and monitoring form used in Functional Medicine to quantify the incidence of symptoms and their frequency. Higher scores are associated with greater toxicity and diminished health. A score of over 100 indicates severe toxicity, 50-100 moderate toxicity, 10-50 mild toxicity, and optimal is less than 10. Helena's first score in 2008 was 188 prior to any nutritional intervention. She was initially put on a modified food elimination diet to remove common antigenic and inflammatory foods along with a 45-day detoxification protocol. Her subsequent weekly scores were 100, 42, and then 23, indicating a trend toward significant improvement in her health status. In addition to a medical food powder designed to support liver detoxification pathways she was given borage oil, EPA/DHA, vitamin A, D3, and C supplements, along with digestive system support of probiotics, immunoglobulins, and a supplement to support the gastrointestinal tract which included L-glutamine, N-Acetyl glucosamine, deglycyrrhizinated licorice, aloe vera leaf, MSM, slippery elm bark, and marshmallow root. Other interventions included the use of anti-inflammatory foods and additional supplements such as boswellia, ginger, and turmeric as needed. Although she did very well on this initial course of nutritional intervention, after a number of months she began to return to former dietary habits and was less regular with her chiropractic and massage therapies. There were additional stressors in her life, including conflict in her primary relationship, and her symptoms either returned, worsened, and/or new symptoms were present.

In 2011 she repeated the MSQ questionnaire with a score of 137. At that time she was placed on an anti-candida protocol for three months followed by a low antigenic anti-inflammatory diet. A similar nutritional protocol was used without the medical food and with the addition of anti-microbial herbs such as berberine or black walnut as well as digestive enzymes with meals. Her subsequent MSQ scores were 78, 43 and 9, once again indicating a trend toward improved health. Her body weight dropped 15 pounds, body fat percentage was 37% and her waist circumference was reduced to 30 inches. This decrease in the physiological active adipose tissue indicates a reduction of inflammatory chemicals. During that time she was more regular with chiropractic care and we added stress management techniques such as diaphragmatic breathing, meditation, and listening to music. She was referred to an acupuncturist to facilitate pain relief and assist in restoration of organ function.

Although it was suggested, Helena was resistant to psychotherapy as a modality to assist with the challenges and change of status in her primary relationship. She was however very motivated to regain strength and continue to improve her body composition. She was referred to a personal trainer where she continued to show improvement in mobility, flexibility, agility and strength as well as experience greater self-confidence and improved energy. As her symptoms began to vastly improve with the program of care and lifestyle changes her frustration with her health issues has diminished but not completely resolved. We needed to educate her on the nature of autoimmune diseases; they are typically managed not cured.

Currently Helena has a greater sense of hope and control over her health and life. She has learned how lifestyle impacts her health and vitality as well as how to use the modalities of chiropractic, nutrition, exercise, massage, and acupuncture to maintain her health and well-being. Ongoing wellness care will encourage continued improvement and management of changes or exacerbations of her condition.

IMPLICATIONS FOR SOCIAL WORK PRACTICE

Integrative Medicine has the potential for unique contributions to people with lupus. As a patient-centered orientation with the relationship between patient and practitioner at its core, IM provides a conceptual model for providing a multidisciplinary approach to care for people with autoimmune diseases such as SLE. The IM approach of Functional Medicine emphasizes this therapeutic partnership which engages the heart, mind, and spirit of both practitioner and client. This partnership encourages a full biopsychosocial assessment and deeper insight into the contributing factors of complex medical problems.

It is important for a social worker to have a basic working understanding of the etiology of autoimmune diseases, the various therapeutic interventions available, including CAM, and the referral sources best suited for each patient. Current research gives valuable insight into the possible factors associated with a dysregulated immune system as well as implications for treatment with natural, less invasive therapies, including diet and lifestyle changes. Social workers can encourage lifestyle changes for their clients to include whole foods, nutrition, movement, stress management, and social support. When patients are able to make positive lifestyle changes with potential to have a positive impact on the quality of their lives, there exists the probability that they may gain some sense of control over their health status, thus providing an opportunity for healing.

CONCLUSION

Social workers and allied health professionals with awareness of Integrative Medicine and CAM approaches are often in the best position to facilitate a holistic integrative approach to the myriad of stress reactions that are commonly experienced by SLE patients. Understanding the reciprocal relationship between biological and psychosocial factors can often provide more effective assessment and treatment, and facilitate the body's natural healing response. In addition to psychosocial interventions, emphasis on lifestyle changes, with referrals to appropriate practitioners when necessary, can have a significant positive impact on the quality of life for people living with lupus.

Although Integrative Medicine providers are cognizant of working with the whole person, including the emotional and mental influences on health status, most do not address the role family and loved ones have in the management of patients with Lupus. Future research can explore the effects that family support or lack of support have on the health status of people with SLE. Additional research may include the relationship between positive lifestyle changes a person with SLE makes in an Integrative Medicine model, how the family system responds to those changes, and what impact the family response has on the long term adherence to beneficial lifestyle modifications.

REFERENCES

Brady, D.M. (2012). Autoimmune Disease: A Modern Epidemic? Molecular Mimicry, the Hygiene Hypothesis, Stealth Infections, and Other Examples of Disconnect Between Medical Research and the Practice of Clinical Medicine. *Townsend Letter, the Examiner of Alternative Medicine.* Retrieved from http://www.townsendletter.com/June2012/autoimmune0612.html [July 28, 2012].

Crosbie, D., Black, C., McIntyre, L., Royle, P., Thomas, S. (2007). Dehydroepiandrosterone for systemic lupus erythematosus. *Cochrane Database of Systematic Reviews*, (4). doi: 10.1002/14651858.CD005114 [pii].

Das, U.N. (2010). Current and emerging strategies for the treatment and management of systemic lupus erythematosus based on molecular signatures. *Journal of Inflammation Research*, (3), 143-170.

Fitzgerald, K. (2011). A Case Report of a 53-Year-Old Female with Rheumatoid Arthritis and Osteoporosis: Focus on Lab Testing and CAM Therapies. *Alternative Medicine Review*, 16(3).

Hoffman, D. (2003). *Medical Herbalism: the science and practice of herbal medicine.* Rochester, VT: Healing Arts Press.

Horrigan, B, Lewis, S, Abrams, D, and Pechura, C. (2012). Integrative Medicine in America: How Integrative Medicine is being practiced in clinical centers across the United States. *The Bravewell Collaborative.*

Jones, D.S. (2006). *Textbook of Functional Medicine.* Gig Harbor, WA: The Institute of Functional Medicine.

Kamhi, E. and Zampieron, E.R. (2006). *Arthritis: Reverse Underlying Causes of Arthritis with Clinically Proven Alternative Therapies* (2nd ed.). Berkeley: Celestial Arts.

Patavino, T. and Brady, D.M. (2001). Natural medicine and nutritional therapy as an alternative treatment in systemic lupus erythematosus. *Alternative Medicine Review*, 6(5), 460-471.

Pender, M.P. (2012). CD8+ T-Cell Deficiency, Epstein-Barr Virus Infection, Vitamin D Deficiency, and Steps to Autoimmunity: A Unifying Hypothesis. *Autoimmune Diseases.* doi:10.1155/2012/189096.

Perandini, L.A., de Sá-Pinto, A.L., Roschel, H., Benatti, F.B., Lima, F.R., Bonfá, E., Gualano, B.Rev. (2012). Jul 7. [Epub ahead of print] Exercise as a therapeutic tool to counteract inflammation and clinical symptoms in autoimmune rheumatic diseases. *Autoimmunity Reviews.* Retrieved at http://dx.doi.org.ezproxy.nycc.edu:2048/10.1016/j.autrev [July 7 2012].

Rakel, D. (2007). *Integrative Medicine* (2nd ed.). Philadelphia, PA: Saunders Elsevier.

Tench, C.M., McCarthy, J., McCurdie I., White, P.D. and D'Cruz, D.P. (2003). Fatigue in systemic lupus erythematosus: a randomized controlled trial of exercise. *Rheumatology.* 42, 1050-1054. doi:10.1093/rheumatology/keg289.

Vickers, A.J., Cronin, A.M., Maschino, A.C., et al. Acupuncture for Chronic Pain: Individual Patient Data Meta-analysis. *Arch Intern Med.* Published online September 10, 2012. doi:10.1001/archinternmed.2012.3654.

http://www.functionalmedicine.org/about/whatisfm/.

http://www.functionalmedicine.org/themovement/in-clinical-practice [retrieved October 5, 2012].

http://www.lifeinthefastlane.com/resources/oslerisms/ [retrieved October 5, 2012].

http://www.nccam.nih.gov/sites/nccam.nih.gov/files/D347_05-25-2012.pdf [retrieved October 5, 2012].

Listening to Lupus Patients and Families: Fine Tuning the Assessment

N. L. BECKERMAN, LCSW, DSW

Wurzweiler School of Social Work, Yeshiva University, New York, New York, USA

MICHELE SARRACCO, LCSW

New York, New York, USA

Given the chronicity and uncertainty of lupus, patients and their family members will face physical, financial, social, and emotional challenges that can be overwhelming. This article records the experiences of three different families affected by lupus. Although these patients and families are very different, their perspectives identify common emotional challenges. Understanding these experiences from their perspectives can help facilitate an assessment that is highly attuned to the potential psychosocial impact of lupus on the patient and the family.

INTRODUCTION

Lupus is a chronic autoimmune disease marked by moderate and sometimes debilitating fatigue, joint inflammation, and potential organ involvement when the patient is in "a flare" (Lupus Foundation of America, 2001; Giffords, 2003; Lindner & Lederman, 2009; Seawell & Danoff-Burg, 2004; Wallace, 2000). Given the chronicity, uncertainty, potential acuity of the disease, and

---

The authors acknowledge the contributions of the three families who generously shared their stories, and the assistance of Karen White, MSW.

treatment side effects that can be difficult to tolerate, the patient and family will face emotional hurdles that can be enduring and arduous (Beckerman, Auerbach, & Blanco, 2011; Danoff-Burg & Friedberg, 2009; Moses, Wiggers, Nicholas, & Cockburn, 2005; Pullen, Brewer, & Ballard, 2009).

Certain emotional challenges for this population have emerged from recent research: the vulnerability to depression and anxiety, coping with changes in appearance, adapting to restricted physical abilities, living with chronic uncertainty and coping with various losses throughout the course of the illness (Adams, Dammers, Saia, Brantley, & Gaydos, 1994; Dobkin, Fortin, Esdaile, Danoff, & Clarke, 1998; Mendelson, 2006; Moses et al., 2005; Sperry, 2009). Based on interviews with three families deeply affected by SLE, this article shares the stories of patients and family members as they describe their respective emotional challenges in their own words. These SLE patients and families were part of a larger qualitative study ($n = 32$) that employed focus group interviews (Beckerman, 2011). In listening to these narratives, the mental health practitioner can better understand the emotional impact of this illness as well as the extraordinary strengths of patients and families as they navigate life with SLE. From these narratives, the practitioner can gain insight into the heart of the emotional challenges posed by lupus and, in turn, can cultivate a more sensitive and effective assessment.

LITERATURE REVIEW: PSYCHOSOCIAL IMPACT FOR THE PATIENT AND FAMILY

There has been growing empirical research identifying the psychosocial experiences and needs of those living with systemic lupus erythematosus (SLE), commonly referred to as lupus in the United States (Giffords, 2003; Mendolson 2006; Seawell & Danoff-Burg, 2004). Psychological distress is common in SLE patients, and anxiety and depression are particularly common (Moses et al., 2005; Seawell & Danoff-Burg, 2004). SLE can cause disturbances of mood such as depression, nervousness, confusion, decreased concentration, and insomnia (Walker et al., 2000). These can be caused by the disease activity itself, the chronic and debilitating nature of the illness, as well as the acute stages of flares (Bauman, Barnes, Schreiber, Dunsmore, & Brooks, 1989; Kulczycka, Sysa-Jedrzejowski, & Robal, 2010; McElhone, Abott, & The, 2006; Moses et al., 2005). The cycle of chronicity and acuity can result in an overall worsening quality of life, both physically and emotionally (Kulczycka et al., 2010).

Moses et al. (2005) developed and employed a Needs Assessment Questionnaire specifically for SLE patients ($n = 386$) and reported that in addition to depression regarding physical limitations, many SLE patients lived with a fear of exacerbation, feelings of depression, anxiety, and stress (Moses et al., 2005, p. 37). Beckerman and colleagues (2011) facilitated a cross-sectional, exploratory study ($n = 378$) of SLE patients to ascertain their unique psychosocial challenges. Among their findings, self-reported depressive and anxious feelings were common for SLE patients; these were primarily due to: (1) changes in appearance due to SLE, (2) limitations in physical abilities (not able to do what they used to do), and (3) medication side effects. These findings concur with Seawell and Danoff-Burg (2005) who identified the impact that lupus-related weight gain, facial rashes, and hair loss can have on the mood and self-esteem of women battling the illness.

Danoff-Burg and Friedberg (2009) studied the unmet psychosocial needs of SLE patients ($n = 112$). Findings indicated that the anxiety and stress involved family relationships, with nearly half ($n = 48\%$) desiring assistance related to maintaining relationships (Danoff-Burg & Friedberg, 2009).

Lindner and Lederman (2009) studied lupus patients ($n = 154$) and found that more than half (56%) were classified as moderate/clinically depressed due to the impact of the disease. The illness itself, physical pain and limitations, medical regimen, and side effects were identified as the sources of depression. Understandably, the worse the symptomotalogy and the more recent the acute lupus flares, the more depressed the sample felt (Lindner & Lederman, 2009).

Kulczycka et al. (2009) studied SLE patients ($n = 83$) and correlated emotional states with the activity and duration of the disease; that is, the more prevalent the symptoms, the more likely patients will experience negative emotions and states of depression (Kululczycka et al. 2009). This is in concurrence with Shorthall, Isenberg, & Newman (1995); Seawell & Danoff-Burg (2004); Rinaldi et al. (2006); and Segui et al. (2000). Interestingly, the converse relationship has been found as Pawlak, Witten, and Heiken (2003) identified that a perceived state of stress can actually trigger a flare.

When a loved one becomes chronically ill, families are confronted with the need to adapt their pre-morbid functional and emotional norms to an illness-centered norm (Sperry, 2009). As they attempt to adapt to the chronic state of uncertainty, often there is marital strain and familial discord (Karlson et al., 2004; Sperry, 2009). Assessment of marital strain in the lives of SLE patients may result in an opportunity to address an unspoken but common stressor for the SLE patient (Karlson et al., 2004). Training on self-efficacy, couple communication skills, social support, and problem solving could ease marital conflict and enhance the couple's ability to cope adaptively with the challenges that SLE might pose for the patient and family (Campbell & Patterson, 1995; Goodman, Morissey, Graham, & Bossingham, 2005; Keller, 1999).

Parental chronic illness can disrupt the family processes and strains both marital intimacies and parent/child relationships (Baider & Spexiele, 1997; Faulkner & Davey, 2002). Additionally, the inability to maintain employment due to SLE, and the expenses of health care and prescriptions can combine to create a series of financial stressors that can result in ongoing conflict for the family (Danoff-Burg & Friedberg, 2009; Tench, McCurdie, White, & D'Cruz, 2000). Karasz and Ouillette (1995) studied women with SLE and found that women with SLE experience acute psychological distress linked to the loss of their valued social roles as wife, mother, sister, daughter, and friend. Other studies concur that role strain is a common theme (Beckerman, 2011; Doria, Rinaldi, & Ermani, 2004; Moses et al., 2005).

THREE FAMILIES AFFECTED BY SLE

Three patients and their significant others (interviewed from a larger qualitative focus groups on the subject) shared how SLE impacted their lives. These three family systems were selected to represent different levels of SLE manifestations (moderate and severe) different family dynamics and different racial, cultural and socioeconomic perspectives. As well, each family demonstrated their own resilience and respective sources of strength in the face of chronic illness.

Susan and Family

Susan is a heavy-set 18-year-old Jamaican teen who lives at home with both her parents and her younger sister. She had just started taking classes at a community college when she experienced sudden acute pains in her knees and ankles. She says she remembers trying to walk up the stairs to her classes and she just was not able to because of the extreme pain in her knees. Days later these pains were accompanied by high fevers and fatigue. During her first hospitalization, there was no definitive diagnosis and Susan was treated with steroids to reduce the inflammation. Several months passed as Susan tried to catch up with school work. She and her family hoped that it had been a viral infection. However, three months later, she experienced the same scenario and during a second hospitalization, Susan received the diagnosis of SLE. She has had several other complications since then, but all were managed successfully enough for her to manage with reliance on steroids (Prednisone) and other anti-inflammatories. She is supported by her parents. Her medication regimen has caused mood changes, anxiety, wakefulness, and weight gain, chiefly a swollen face. Her health care insurance is provided by her parents and there are numerous conflicts regarding the financial strain; primarily paying for her SLE medication co-payments. Susan is able to manage in the apartment and in her neighborhood, but avoids any transportation that includes stairs. The weight gain from her steroids was particularly upsetting for Susan, who had been trying to reduce her weight through her teen years and had just achieved her weight goal prior to the onset of SLE. "It was just so defeating. No matter how hard I try now, I can't take off weight and I have this fat face. Who's going to want to date me?"

When asked about her most challenging moments, Susan said that she felt that while she could make every effort to stay healthy with nutrition, exercise, enough rest and preventive care, she found herself, "always waiting, always waiting for the first signal that my body is in trouble and that she is going to have another flare." She added, "I'd like to go back to school and pursue my education, but I just don't know if it's realistic. I keep trying to get it under control, but I don't know if there's such a thing." When asked how she has coped with these thoughts and feelings, she answered,

> I have no control. Maybe I never did, but now I really know it. That's what I learned. Each day I have that I'm not ill is a big relief. I try to be optimistic and hope that if I make plans, I'll be healthy enough when that day comes. If I'm not, I hope others will understand. The fatigue I feel isn't like the flu, it's like I've been knocked over by a bus. I just try to remind myself that I have a good family, and that people have it worse. I have to think I'm lucky that I have my family to depend on.

Susan also shared that she attends a monthly support group and other events for SLE patients at her SLE clinic. "This is a great comfort to me. Talking to other SLE patients has been so helpful. Only they know what it's like to have the disease, to feel too tired to get out of bed, to feel pain in your joints. I've talked to my family, but I already rely on them so much, particularly when I'm sick, I don't like to upset my parents or my sister." Susan's positive experience through her affiliation to her lupus group is an example of what Ng et al. (2007) found when they reported that a lupus support group can be a primary source of support in enhancing the psychological well-being for a lupus patient.

Family Perspectives

Susan's parents and her sister explained that they were shocked by her diagnosis. They had never heard of lupus and were still learning about it. They have tried to be as supportive as possible, but all work full time and her younger sister is in high school and works part time. "It's not easy because we all have other obligations . . . and also we don't want to upset her . . . and always asking her how she feels." They have tried to carry on as normally as possible, and have also tried to be available to her when she is in a flare. When asked if they could identify their most difficult emotional challenge, Susan's parents explained that they want her to be hopeful and live a normal life, but they are always worried for her. "I worry all the time. She was so sick, we were afraid we were going to lose her. I worry that the next time it will be her kidneys or heart. What if she can't find a loving man or keep her job. It's a terrible time to be out of work." Her dad finished by saying, "The biggest upset is seeing her in pain and feeling so helpless."

In addition to coping with loss and uncertainty, Susan's family showed us a common dynamic for families faced with chronic illness; the patient is trying to shield her family from upset and her family is trying to protect the patient from their upset. Several studies in chronic illness report that this dynamic can increase emotional distancing just when family members may need emotional intimacy the most (Beckerman, 2006).

Nic and Her Mother

Nic is a 33-year-old African-American, Baptist woman, living with her mother and her 14- year-old son. Nic is wheelchair-bound, has lost vision in her left eye, and is taking numerous medications for cardiac and heart damage as a result of her SLE. She lives in a small apartment, receives Public Assistance, Social Security Disability (SSD), and is covered by Medicaid. The raised thresholds between each room in the apartment were taken up so that Nic can navigate her wheelchair from room to room, but she is not able to enter the kitchen because the wheelchair cannot be accommodated. Her mother has been her primary caregiver. She can navigate around her neighborhood in the wheelchair with her mother's assistance, but she has tremendous difficulty venturing out without a caretaker. Her 14-year-old son returned to her life and is now part of caring for his mother.

When Nic was 10 years old she seemed to bruise easily, experience swelling joints, fevers, and fatigue. Initially, Nic and her mother were told these symptoms might be Rheumatoid Arthritis or Leukemia. Nic had numerous hospitalizations over a period of 18 months with no further clarity. After another battery of tests and examinations by her treating rheumatologist, Nic was diagnosed with lupus. Nic and her mother were told there would be occasional flares of joint pain and fatigue. Neither felt they were fully informed about the range of SLE manifestations, treatment side effects, or potential hazards.

As a teenager, Nic experienced less frequent flares, but the flares she had were life-threatening. At 19, she became pregnant and had a son (1 month premature). During the pregnancy, Nic experienced many serious complications due to lupus and suffered a stroke, lost sight in one eye, and has had ongoing double vision. After giving birth to her son (who was healthy), she was unable to provide primary care because she was so ill and disabled. Her sister took Nic's baby and shared caretaking responsibilities with Nic's mother. Through those early years, Nic had several acute flares marked by cardiac and kidney damage, underwent physical and occupational therapy, transfusions, changes in medial regimens, and ultimately stabilized. She was never able to work again and for most of her son's young life, she visited with him, but other family members shared childrearing responsibilities. When asked how she managed trying to parent with her illness, Nic said: "I go crawling to get to his school or to hear him sing in church. And I spend any shred of energy I have to look after him. He gives me my medicine and I look out for him. We look after each other."

All of this Nic shared with a smile and went on, "I do the best I can. I have my old friends, but they can't handle my illness. My heartbreak is my best friend. She just cannot tolerate seeing me when I'm sick. I know she cares, but she just can't see me in the hospital. That hurts." After a serious flare, Nic was upset about her friend and went to a social worker "to talk things over with someone outside of the family." She was looking for encouragement, she said, or reassurance, and found that most of the questions she was asked were about suicide. "Being a religious woman, I never considered suicide and the worker just asked what she wanted to. I was turned off to social work and never returned."

FAMILY PERSPECTIVES

Frances, Nic's mother, listened to Nic and seemed to agree with all that her daughter had shared. She added that her daughter's health has been the primary activity in her life since Nic's lupus diagnosis. According to her, they are "best friends" and can intuit each other's moods and needs. Her life has been centered on Nic's medical appointments (rheumatologist, nephrologist, and cardiologist) and the two have become inseparable. When asked how that has affected her life, Frances answered, "Sometimes I want to go out somewhere, but my daughter can't, so I don't want to go and leave her." She expanded that she felt "caught" between feeling she should be with her daughter and wanting "some space" to herself outside of her daughter's illness. In her belief, she could only be as independent as her daughter's condition allowed. She explained that as her daughter has lost her independence, so too, has she. When she did venture into activities that were unrelated to her daughter, she experienced too much guilt and remorse to enjoy herself.

Regarding the uncertainty in their lives, Frances felt that she was "always on call and always on edge." Frances lives each day with a sense of anxiety about any changes in Nic. If her daughter expresses any fluctuation in her physical status, both mother and daughter fear that this could be a warning signal that the "lupus is flaring." She provided a poignant metaphor of a lupus flare when she explained, "It's like no matter how many locks we put on the door, you hear a noise and you never know when that door's going to be broken down."

Frances has turned to good girlfriends she says she can talk to about the stresses of Nic's illness. When asked what has been most helpful, both mother and adult daughter expressed a very deep faith that they have relied on for strength and solace throughout the course of Nic's illness.

Mr. P.

Mr. P., a White male professional educator in his late sixties who was asked to describe the psychosocial experiences he has had with his wife who has had SLE for several decades. They have private insurance and have experienced financial strain, but have been able to adapt to these financial stressors adequately. His wife was too ill to participate. In his own words, "I should make clear that the voyage is always a combination of universal and personal responses since the experience is dependent on the relationship between the partners and the many different physical manifestations that lupus can take." This is his perception, distinct from his wife's perceptions of how lupus has affected their lives. Mr. P. explained that in dealing with SLE, "it can best be categorized as having had three phases. They are: facing an unknown condition, active lupus phase and living with uncertainty."

DIAGNOSIS—FACING AN UNKNOWN CONDITION

In the first phase, at the age of 32 (1971), his wife had significant joint pain that made it difficult for her to work. In retrospect, they realized that earlier pulmonary problems, fatigue, and some false positives on tests were due to lupus. In reviewing her various symptoms, Mr. and Mrs. P. were later able to date her lupus onset back to age 19. "However, in 1971, this was no longer a manageable situation, but a significant problem; the search for what the medical problem was began." Mr. P. explained, "Some days were better than others, but her fatigue meant that she went to bed early and due to the stiffness in her joints she had difficulty getting up in the morning and was sometimes crippled by her joint pain." With three young sons at the time, they tried to create and maintain a normal situation and Mr. P. found himself trying to protect his wife from the demands of family life. There were repeated visits to different physicians and repeated medical tests, which were of no help in identifying the cause of her condition. "For me, there was a sense of frustration and failure that there was nothing I could do." The physicians seemed to agree that while she had many lupus symptoms she did not have SLE since the "tests" for SLE were negative. She recovered without an official diagnosis.

ACTIVE LUPUS PHASE

Mrs. P. experienced several years without a significant relapse. However, while traveling, Mrs. P experienced a chest cold and was treated with antibiotics. Despite treatment, her condition worsened. Mr. P. said that in retrospect, "her condition was probably exacerbated by antibiotics. As with many lupus patients, she has allergies to many antibiotics." Mr. P explained that "at this point, she had a raft of SLE symptoms including traveling joint pains and the telltale facial rash, but the definitive lupus test was negative."

Mr. P struggled with advocating for his wife "to break through the medical stonewall and get the doctors to treat her for lupus." Mr. P's experience with the barrage of physicians was primarily negative and he took it upon himself to research the test for SLE. Subsequently, he discovered this test had substantial false negative rates. He pressed this issue with a physician who then began to treat his wife for SLE. She was in a critical state during this lupus flare. At this time, Mr. P. had just begun the stressors of a new job, was trying to help one son off to college, and was providing, as best as he could, a home life for the other two younger sons.

It was several more weeks before his wife was strong enough to be discharged. "It was clear that she could not be left alone, so I arranged for someone to come in during the day when I was not home." Mr. P. recalls that his wife was "very weak and her main activity was being sure to get dressed so the children would not see her still in her night clothes when they came home."

> The life of our children was radically changed. There was the question of what do you tell the children? But how do you provide reassurance when you are not even sure yourself about what the future will be like. Certainly, once she was at home I placed more demands on them not to make a lot of noise. I felt guilty about that since they were just being normal kids.

Mr. P. explained that he wanted to encourage her independence, but also had to accept and contend with realistic limitations created by his wife's lupus. He understood she should not be left alone while convalescing, but he needed to go out to do errands. However, when he did go out, he felt that his wife experienced his actions as a type of desertion. Not to upset her while she was ill, he remained at home, but felt trapped by the situation. Eventually, after several trial voyages together, Mrs. P. was somewhat more confident to venture out with her husband. As he explained, "Given the oversized part that the illness plays and the need to protect what energy one's partner has, one has a tendency to withdraw from one's broader social network of friends." Mr. P. spoke of the balance between the reality of the illness and its limitations; realizing life is no longer what it was prior to the lupus, but trying not to define his partner by her illness.

Mr. and Mrs. P. have weathered several decades with great uncertainty as to the progression of her lupus. There were long periods with manageable lupus symptoms and several acute flares. According to Mr. P., in most flares, they were able to suppress the severity with medication regimens.

> Given the uncertainty, the occasional joint pains and fatigue, she has never returned to work. You come to realize that lupus will be forever a part of your life together. There are places in the world where

you will never go because of the high risks associated with not having readily available medical care or the strenuous conditions one would face. We have had to have a wait and see attitude about what it will be possible to do.

Mr. P. returned to his delicate balance of "supporting his wife's effort to expand the quality of her life and also to be patient if she's not feeling well." Finally, he explained that they had had ups and downs, and that there were times of normalcy, and times when they were particularly fearful it might all start again. Two years later, Mrs. P. experienced another debilitating flare that incapacitated her again for months. This underscored that one "is always living on the edge." He explained that they coped with the ambiguity surrounding her illness by trying to communicate openly with one another and Mrs. P.'s doctors. Mr. P. added that he tried to be patient and tried to enjoy as much normalcy of their married and family life as he could.

DISCUSSION

The three lupus narratives are distinctly different from one another, but there are shared psychosocial challenges. Regardless of whether the illness strikes in adolescence, young adulthood, or later in life, the recurring themes entail coping with loss (present and anticipated) and great uncertainty throughout the course of the illness. The lupus diagnosis enters into the lives of individuals and families with largely unknown consequences, remaining both mysterious and threatening to the emotional and functional well-being of all members. The functional and emotional norms will have to shift to adapt to the disease manifestations, the chronicity, acuity, and the potential of reoccurrence of illness.

As noted in the literature and illustrated in the case studies, there are two broad themes that pose psychosocial challenges for lupus patient and their families:

- **Loss** (including loss of some physical capabilities, anticipatory loss, loss of identity, loss of family equilibrium, loss of independence)
- **Coping with Uncertainty** (unknown course of illness, changing physical capabilities, medication side effects, how others will react, if others will understand)

Loss

For the individual living with lupus, there may be various dimensions of functional losses as well as current or anticipated emotional losses to navigate. For Susan, as she struggled to maintain her weight while on Prednisone, she spoke of a loss of self-esteem, and "loss of control over my weight." Nic had significant physical losses and because of the subsequent limitations, she endured the loss of her role as a mother and loss of freedom to socialize with her friends. As she explained, "I just wanted to take care of my son and hang out with my friends and do normal things, but I wasn't able to." Mr. P. experienced the loss of his wife as an "active participant" and the loss of "a sense of normalcy of family life."

In addition to the functional challenges the family may face, they have had to navigate feelings about losses that have occurred and the anticipated losses that may not have occurred yet; a dynamic referred to as ambiguous loss (Boss, 1999). The ways in which these feelings are expressed and navigated in the family relationships is a central area of assessment for the mental health practitioner. Mr. P. describes this in his moving metaphor of the "dreaded" return of "the sword of Damocles" that is always in the "back of one's mind" and keeps one "always living on the edge."

In the family affected by lupus, the practitioner can also assess for the level of tension around loss of independence (for both patient and family members) and how that tension is experienced and navigated. In the above cases, one can see that Susan has had to cope with a sense of diminished independence as she has had to rely on her family to help her cope at a time she was about to pursue a college education that would have launched her into autonomy. Likewise, her family has had to deal with her increased dependency needs and possible loss of their own sense of freedom as so pointedly expressed by her sister, "I want her to know she can always count on me, but I also want to live my own life." Similarly, in the case of Nic, her mother expressed the same sense of loss of her own autonomy in the face of her daughter's illness when she stated that she wants "to go out somewhere, but my daughter can't, so I don't want to go and leave her." For Mr. P., while contending with the losses caused by his wife's lupus, he struggled with loss of his own independence. As these cases have revealed, the patient and family attempt to balance the wish to lead "normal" lives while accepting the reality of the losses and limitations that lupus has created.

In the face of these current and potential losses, assessment should focus on how the individual and family have attempted to cope, with an emphasis on identifying preexisting coping styles and current coping abilities. Assessment should seek to explore the past emotional challenges or dyadic conflicts that may be triggered by the illness or is a direct reaction to the illness. A family assessment around this theme of loss and its adaptations may provide an opportunity to share emotional reactions and reestablish those functional interactions that serve the family well (Goodman et al., 2005).

Coping With Uncertainty

Although the concept of uncertainty is one that might apply to any chronic illness with an unclear course, it is clearly a prevailing emotional challenge for those coping with lupus. This primary issue has been identified in each of the cases that have been presented. Uncertainty begins at the onset of the diagnostic phase as one is "facing an unknown condition" and continues to dominate throughout the course of the illness. The prevalence and the psychosocial impact of uncertainty is so imposing that Mr. P chose to classify living with lupus as "living with uncertainty."

Lupus presents patients and loved ones with a dual universe of emotions; coping with the present illness and living with a great anxiety about if and when the illness will flare again (Boss, 1999; Moses et al., 2005). Continual exposure to uncertainty can alter the functional and emotional interplay of the family as well as the developmental milestones of each family member. These levels of uncertainty have a corrosive effect on spousal intimacy and relationship stability, resulting in higher rates of marital discord, separation, and divorce among those living with lupus (Sperry, 2009). The experience of a chronic illness such as lupus can create a certain existential insecurity and this emotional experience can be exacerbated when the disorder is hard to diagnose, likely to be chronic, and often involves the disruption of a previously projected life plan (Stockl, 2007).

This was exemplified in Susan's narrative when she stated she would "like to go back to school and pursue my education, but I just don't know if it's realistic." Similarly, this was evidenced by Nic who shared that, "I never know if what I'm feeling is the beginning of a flare." Mr. P grappled with uncertainty and asked: "How do you provide reassurance when you are not even sure yourself about what the future will be like?"

In each of these families there were extraordinary internal and external strengths to be found. Stockl (2007) points out that when facing an uncertain illness, most people find themselves driven to gather a considerable amount of expert knowledge about their condition that turns them into a "proto-professional" (Stockl, 2007). Susan's efforts to stay healthy by informing herself about nutrition, exercise, and preventive care would therefore be encouraged as strength in her efforts to cope. Likewise, Mr. P's researching the test for lupus qualifies him as being a "proto-professional" in an attempt to deal with the sense of uncertainty. Susan's efforts to educate herself about her illness, her participation in her support group, and her positive outlook were notable strengths and signs of resilience. Nic and her mother's reliance on their religion proved great sources of emotional and functional support. All three families exhibited resourcefulness, inner strength, and resilience in the face of loss and uncertainty.

ASSESSMENT IMPLICATIONS

It is important to assess what the patient and family know about the illness and how they have tried to cope and adapt before pursuing more complex emotional challenges. As Karlson et al. (2004) noted, the biopsychosocial framework is essential in counseling lupus patients and their families, and therefore the development of any assessment should be based on the understanding that the systemic impact of such an illness will reverberate on multiple levels. A dynamic assessment should include the ways in which the uncertainty and loss surrounding the illness may have impeded intimacy, obstructed the developmental individual and family stages or shifted the family's equilibrium. As well, the assessment should seek to identify and facilitate adaptive adjustments that the family can rely on to manage the pervasive uncertainty and loss in the system.

Whether you are counseling an individual, a dyad, or the family system, the impact of loss and coping with uncertainty can be assessed with attention to the interdependence of the individual and his/her family. It is important to look at what the strengths and challenges of the system are/have been and how to support the functional patterns of coping or the development of new coping abilities in place of those that were maladaptive (Saleebey, 2002). When there are children impacted by a parents' chronic illness, one dimension of assessment should include the social role re-alignment around the illness that may interrupt normative development. While Nic might "go crawling to get to his school" can be seen as an inner strength that needs to be capitalized on, the social worker should also consider the potential for enmeshed boundaries and parentified children in the face of illness. The stage of illness, the patient and family's unique motivation capacity and opportunity for engaging in counseling will dictate which theoretical frameworks will be most effective (Ripple, Ernestina, & Polemis, 1964). Medical family therapy, crisis-intervention, cognitive-behavioral, and emotionally focused theories have all been used effectively in assisting a family facing the psychosocial impact of a medical illness (Boss & Couden, 2002; Campbell & Patterson, 1995; Rinaldi et al., 2006). Early in diagnosis or in an acute flare, there is room to rely on crisis intervention to help the family unit to cope with initial shock and anxiety and to re-establish functional and emotional equilibrium. As patients and families begin to adapt, family therapy, cognitive, and emotional approaches may have more traction (Boss & Couden, 2002; Campbell & Patterson, 1995).

As always with a patient facing chronic medical illness, assessment should include the nature of the relationship SLE patients have with their health care providers and previous social workers. In the above cases, social work was not a central component of care. Only Nic met with a social worker to discuss the psychosocial impact of her illness, and unfortunately that was a negative experience. Susan and Mrs. P. commented that a social worker may have interviewed them while they were hospitalized, but they could not recall anything significant from that interaction. The one resounding positive relationship with social work was for Susan, who had a very affirmative relationship with her group and the social worker who facilitated these sessions. Faced with the diagnosis of a serious and life alter-ing chronic illness, there should be an automatic and comprehensive social work assessment as part of health care provision and planning.

CONCLUSION

This article reviewed the perspectives of three different families regarding how they were affected by lupus. These perspectives were used as a means of identifying the key emotional challenges to individuals and families who are facing this diagnosis in order to provide effective assessments. In the process of listening to their stories, the experiences of loss and uncertainty were identified across the three narratives. How these themes manifested and how the patient and family attempted to cope with these emotional challenges was highlighted. It is through active and sensitive listening for these themes that we can truly arrive at a deeper understanding of both the emotional pain and the extraordinary strength that takes place while patients and families cope with a chronic illness such as lupus. Most importantly, careful listening can reveal a palpable guide toward a deeper understanding of living with this chronic illness, as in Frances' metaphor: "It's like no matter how many locks we put on the door, you hear a noise and you never know when that door's going to be broken down."

REFERENCES

Adams, S.G., Dammers, P.M., Saia, T.L. Brantley, P.J., & Gaydos, G.R. (1994). Stress, depression and anxiety predict average symptom severity and daily symptom fluctuation in SLE. *Journal of Behavioral Medicine, 17*, 459–477.

Baider, R., & Spexiele, B.A. (1997). Couples' sexual intimacy and MS. *Journal of Family Psychotherapy, 8*(1), 13–22.

Bauman, A., Barnes, C., Schreiber, L., Dunsmore, J., & Brooks, P. (1989). The unmet needs of patients with Systemic Lupus Erythematosus; Planning for patient education. *Patient Education, Patient Educational Counseling, 14*(4), 235–242.

Beckerman, N.L. (2006). *Couples of mixed HIV status: Clinical issues and interventions.* Binghamton, NY: Haworth Press.

Beckerman, N.L. (2011). Living with lupus: A qualitative report. *Social Work in Health Care, 50*(4), 330–343.

Beckerman, N.L., Auerbach, C., & Blanco, I. (2011). Psychosocial dimensions of SLE: Implications for the health care team. *Multidisciplinary Journal of Health Care, 2011*(4), 67–72.

Boss, P. (1999). Ambiguous loss. In F. Walsh & M. McGoldrick (Eds.), *Living beyond loss: Death in the family* (pp. 237–246). New York, NY: W.W. Norton & Company, Inc.

Boss, P., & Couden, B. (2002). *Ambiguous loss from chronic physical illness: clinical interventions with individuals, couples, and families.* New York, NY: Wiley Periodicals, Inc.

Campbell, T., & Patterson, J. (1995). The effectiveness of family interventions in treatment of physical illness. *Journal of Marital and Family Therapy, 21*(4), 543–583.

Danoff-Burg, S., & Friedberg, F. (2009). Unmet needs of patients with SLE. *Behavioral Medicine, 35*(1), 5–14.

Dobkin, P., Fortin, P.R., Joseph, L., Esdaile, J.M., Danoff, D.S, & Clarke, A.E. (1998). Psychosocial contributors to mental and physical health in patients with SLE. *Arthritis Care Research, 11*, 23–31.

Doria, A., Rinaldi, S., & Ermani, M. (2004). Health-related quality of life in Italian patients with systemic lupus erythematosus II. Role of clinical, immunological and psychological determinants. *Rheumatology, 43*, 1580–1586.

Faulkner, R.A., & Davey, M. (2002). Children and adolescents of cancer patients: The impact of cancer on the family. *American Journal of Family Therapy, 30*(1), 63–72.

Giffords, E. (2003). Understanding and managing systemic lupus erythematosus (SLE). *Social Work in Health Care, 37*(4), 57–72.

Goodman, D., Morrissey, S., Graham, D. & Bossingham, D. (2005). The application of cognitive-behaviour therapy in altering illness representations of systemic lupus erythematosus. *Behaviour Change, 22*, 156–171.

Karasz, A., & Ouillette, S. (1995). Role strain and psychological well-being in women with systemic lupus erythematosus. *Women in Health, 23*, 41–57.

Karlson, E., Liang, M., Eaton, H., Huang, J., Fitzgerald, L., Rogers, M., & Daltroy, L. (2004). A randomized clinical trial of a psychoeducational intervention to improve outcomes in systemic lupus erythematosus. *Arthritis & Rheumatism, 50*, 1832–1841.

Keller, S.M. (1999). Social support and psychological distress in women with systemic lupus erythematosus [dissertation]. Ann Arbor, MI: Case Western Reserve University.

Kulczycka, L., Sysa-Jedrzejowska, A., & Robak, E. (2010). Quality of life and satisfaction with life in SLE patients—The importance of clinical manifestations. *Clinical Rheumatology, 29* (9), 991–7.

Lindner, H., & Lederman, L. (2009). Relationship of illness perceptions with depression among individuals diagnosed with lupus. *Depression & Anxiety, 26*(6), 575–582.

Lupus Foundation of America, INC. (2001). Fact Sheet. Lupus Foundation of America, Inc. Retrieved from http://www.lupus.org/education/factsheet.html

McElhone, K., Abbott, J., & The, L.S. (2006). A review of health related quality of life in systemic lupus erythematosus. *Lupus, 15*, 633–643.

Mendelson, C. (2006). Managing a medically and socially complex life: Women living with Lupus. *Qualitative Health Research, 16*(7), 982–997.

Moses, N., Wiggers, J., Nicholas, C., & Cockburn, J. (2005). Prevalence and correlates of perceived unmet needs of people with systemic lupus erythematosus. *Patient Education Counseling, 57*(1), 30–38.

Ng Petrus-Chan, W. (2007). Group psychosocial program for enhancing psychological well-being of people with systemic lupus erythematosus. *Lupus*, 6(3), 75–87.

Pawlak, L.R., Witte, T., & Heiken, H. (2003). Flares in patients with systemic lupus erythematosus are associated with daily psychological stress. *Psychotherapy Psychosomatics*, *72*, 159–165.

Pullen, R., Brewer, S., & Ballard, A. (2009). Putting a face on systemic lupus erythematosus. *Nursing*, *39*(8), 22–33.

Rinaldi, S., Ghisi, M., Iaccarino, L., Zampieri, S., Girardello, A., Piercarlo, S., & Doria, A. (2006). Influence of coping skills on health-related quality of life in patients with Systemic Lupus Erythematosus. *Arthritis & Rheumatism*, *55*, 427–433.

Ripple, L., Ernestina, A., & Polemis, B. (1964). *Motivation, capacity and opportunity*. Chicago, IL: Chicago University Press.

Saleebey, D. (2002). *The Strengths Perspective in Social Work Practice* (3rd ed.). New York, NY: Allyn & Bacon.

Seawell, A.H., & Danoff-Burg, S. (2004). Psychosocial research on SLE: A literature review. *Lupus*, *13*(12), 891–899.

Seawell, A., & Danoff-Burg, S. (2005). Body image and sexuality in women with and without Systemic Lupus Erythematosus. *Sex Roles*, *53*(11–12), 865–876.

Segui, J., Ramos-Casals, M., Garcia-Carrasco, M., de Flores, T., Cerver, R., Valdes, M., & Ingelmo, M. (2000). Psychiatric and psychological disorders in patients with systemic lupus erythematosus: A longitudinal study of active and inactive stages of the disease. *Lupus*, *9*, 584–588.

Shorthall, E., Isenberg, D., & Newman, S. (1995). Factors associated with mood and mood disorders in SLE. *Lupus*, *4*, 272–279.

Sperry, L. (2009). *Treatment of chronic medical conditions*. Washington, DC: American Psychological Association.

Stockl, A. (2007). Complex syndromes, ambivalent diagnosis and existential uncertainty: The case of SLE. *Social Science and Medicine*, *65* (7), 1549–1559.

Tench, C.M., McCurdie, I., White, P.D., & D'Cruz, D.P. (2000). The prevalence and associations of fatigue in SLE, *Rheumatology*, *39*, 1249–1254.

Walker, S., Smarr, K., Parker, J., Weidensaul, D., Nelson, W., & McMurray, R. (2000). Mood states and disease activity in patients with systemic lupus erythematosus treated with bromocriptine. *Lupus*, *9*, 527–533.

Wallace, D.J. (2000). *The lupus book*. New York, NY: Oxford University Press.

Locus of Control and Lupus: Patients' Beliefs, Perspectives, and Disease Activity

CHARLES AUERBACH, MSW, PhD
and N. L. BECKERMAN, LCSW, DSW
Wurzweiler School of Social Work, Yeshiva University,
New York, New York, USA

Patients with lupus often experience a high degree of psychological symptoms such as anxiety, depression, and mood disorders that can influence their beliefs and perceptions of their illness. The purpose of the study was to examine how a patient's self-reported psychosocial needs (depression and anxiety) and beliefs about how much control they have over their health (health locus of control) influences their perception of disease chronicity and acuity. The study findings were based on a survey of 378 patients self-diagnosed with lupus.

INTRODUCTION

Systemic lupus erythematosus (SLE) is a chronic autoimmune disease with acute periodic flares often referred to as lupus. The range of symptoms typically include significant fatigue, joint and muscle pain, dermatological rashes, and in acute events, life-threatening complications due to heart and kidney damage (Rahman & Isenberg, 2008; Wallace, 2000). The existing medications are "powerful and yet imprecise," and in many circumstances, the medical treatments employed in ongoing management "are often as damaging as the disease itself" (Pierce, 2008, p. A11). Disease manifestations, unexpected exacerbations, adverse medication side effects, and disfiguring body changes are often identified as the sources of psychological distress that color one's perception of his/her illness (Danoff-Burg & Friedberg, 2009; Kuriya, Gladman, Ibañez, & Urowitz, 2008; Pons-Estel, Alarcon, Scofield, Reinlib, & Cooper, 2010). This empirical cross-sectional study ($N = 378$) explores the relationship between patient beliefs about their illness and how these beliefs may influence their perceptions of disease activity.

LITERATURE REVIEW

A myriad of psychosocial factors influence the ways in which a patient perceives their own health and illness. There are complex variables such as socioeconomic demographics, the disease manifestation itself, treatment side effects, pre-morbid psychological and emotional functioning, as well as social stressors that all combine to color the level of control a lupus patient feels they have over their illness (Bertoli et al., 2007; Jolly & Utset, 2004; McElhone, Abbott, & Teh, 2009).

In the realm of psychosocial factors; illness perceptions play an important role. Illness perceptions pertain to the beliefs patients develop about their illness. What individuals believe about their level of control over their health and illness will impact their perceptions of the disease activity, their self-management of disease and the emotional sequelae of living with lupus (Babul et al., 2011; Giffords, 2003; Stevens, Hamilton, & Wallston, 2011). Patients with lupus often experience a high degree of psychological symptoms such as anxiety, depression, and mood disorders that can influence their beliefs and perceptions of their illness (Lindner & Lederman, 2009; Monaghan et al., 2007; Moses, Wiggers, Nicholas, & Cockburn, 2005; Bachen, Chesney, & Criswell, 2009; Kozora, Ellison, Waxmonsky, Wamboldt, & Patterson, 2005; Seawell & Danoff-Berg, 2004). There are numerous studies, both empirical and anecdotal, that indicate that lupus patients who feel overwhelmed by the chronicity and uncertainty of the illness are at a high risk for self-reported feelings of depression and anxiety as they cope with the ongoing challenges of this illness (Bachen et al., 2009; Beckerman, Auerbach, & Blanco, 2011; Danoff-Burg and Friedberg, 2004; Khanna, Pandey, & Handa, 2004; Kulczycka, Sysa-Jedrzejowska, & Robak, 2010; Lindner & Lederman, 2009; Monaghan et al., 2007; Moses et al., 2005; Shorthall, Isenberg, & Newman, 1995; Wang, Mayo, & Fortin, 2001).

The complex nature of the bi-directional relationship between emotional states and lupus activity remains inconclusive. In fact while some studies suggest that lupus-related depression may be a result of disease activity, other studies suggest the converse; that depression might have a causative role in triggering an acute flare via the secretion of stress hormones that have shown to accelerate disease activity (Dobkin et al., 1998; Dobkin,

DaCosta, & Fortin, 2001; Iverson, 1992; Seguí et al., 2000; Duvdevany, Cohen Minsker-Valtzer, & Lorber, 2011; Robles, Glaser, Kiecolt-Glaser, 2005).

While several small, qualitative studies with limited ability to generalize have looked at the quality of life for SLE patients, few have directly explored the relationship between illness perceptions and the course of illness (Daleboudt, Broadbent, Berger, & Kaptein, 2011; Goodman, Morrissey, Graham, 2005; Nowicka-Sauer, 2007). Nowicka-Sauer (2007) employed the Illness Perception Questionnaire Revised (IPQ-R), to investigate whether a cognitive behavior therapy (CBT) intervention would influence patients' illness perceptions. The results demonstrated that CBT had indeed influenced and shifted patients' perceptions of their lupus treatment control, as well as the effect of lupus on their emotions (Nowicka-Sauer, 2007).

Goodman et al. (2005) developed and tested a cognitive and behavioral-based intervention ($n = 36$) that demonstrated that interventions that enhance a patient's beliefs that treatments for lupus are effective, resulted in an overall reduction of negative emotional states and overall stress. The more a patient perceived control over their lupus, the less they suffered from both emotional and physical manifestations of lupus. This study indicated that CBT might provide significant improvement in emotional states irrespective of the activity level of the disease (Goodman et al., 2005).

McElhone, Abbott, Gray, Williams, and Teh (2010) aimed to identify and clarify the perspectives of SLE patients ($n = 30$)and how the disease impacted their lives They found that most patients reported a negative impact of SLE on their lives and identified the most relevant themes in their perspectives. Many of these themes concur with the findings of Beckerman et al. (2011); "prognosis and course of disease; body image; effects of treatment; emotional difficulties; inability to plan due to disease unpredictability" (McElhone et al., 2010, p. 1647). These perspectives on their illness resulted in a range of negative emotions, including self-reported feelings of depression. The relationship between a patient's perception of his disease and disease activity is of critical importance (Carr, Nicassion, & Ishimori, 2011). Those with lupus who are emotionally or cognitively negative about their lupus; they are likely to report worsening symptoms, and are three times at risk for treatment non-adherence (DiMatteo, Lepper, & Croghan, 2000; Nery et al., 2007). Given the evidence that there is a significant correlation between a patient's belief about their lupus and their subsequent emotional reactions, self-management and treatment adherence, patients may be at a risk for distorting their symptomatology. The purpose of the study was to examine how a patient's self-reported psychosocial needs (depression and anxiety) and beliefs about how much control they have over their health (health locus of control) influences their perception of disease chronicity and acuity.

METHODOLOGY

Participants and Procedures

All 899 individuals in the S.L.E. Lupus Foundation in New York's contact database received the survey instrument. All patients have been self-diagnosed with SLE. The survey instrument was written at an eighth-grade reading level and was also available in Spanish. The survey was completely anonymous and de-identified. An informed letter was sent along with each survey that explained the purpose of the study, its voluntary nature, that they could discontinue without any penalty and that the information would be used in the aggregate with no identifying information. Packets were distributed by the Foundation to home mailing addresses with stamped envelopes so that completed surveys could be bulk mailed to the researchers at Yeshiva University with complete anonymity. Out of the 880 received, a total of 378 individuals responded for an overall return rate of 42.9%.

Instrument

The survey instrument consisted of three components. Part 1 included sociodemographic variables such as gender, race, and age, length of diagnosis, education, employment, and relationship status. Part 2 consisted of the Systemic Lupus Erythematosus Needs Questionnaire (SLENQ). SLENQ was developed on the basis of the results of a literature review of psychosocial needs associated with having SLE by Moses et al. (2005). The questionnaire was found to be reliable and valid. The SLENQ subscale has been validated, with higher scores reflecting higher need for assistance with self-reported feelings of depression, anxiety, and socioeconomic coping associated with lupus.

Part 3 was the Multidimensional Health Locus of Control Scale (MHLOC) (Wallston & DeVellis, 1978), which measured respondents' beliefs about how much control they have over their health. When patients report that the locus of control is perceived to lie outside of their control, they demonstrate a higher vulnerability to emotional distress (Grotz, Hapke, Lampert, & Baumeister 2011). The MHLOC has demonstrated this to be true for patients facing normative life challenges such as childbirth and aging, as well as a range of chronic health conditions such as high cholesterol, high blood pressure, chronic pancreatitis, and chronic rheumatologic diseases (Pereira, Araújo, Sampaio, & Haddad, 2011; Grotz et al., 2011).

The MHLOC measures the respondents' subjective perceptions of how much control they have over their SLE. Two sub-scales, "Chance" and "Internal," were utilized in this research. "Chance" refers to the mindset that the course of one's illness is out of one's control. "Internal" refers to the opposite perspective; "if I manage my illness with diet, exercise, compliance with medication regimens, I can control its' course." Each is a 6- item self-report questionnaire that uses a 6-point Likert scale with items ranging from 1 = disagree very much to 6 = agree very much. Examples of items included in the chance sub-scale are: "No matter what I do, I am going to get sick," and "Most things that affect my health happen to me by accident." Examples of items included in the internal sub-scale are: "If I get sick, it is my own behavior which determines how soon I get well again" and "I am in control of my health." It is important to note that the sub-scales are independent of each other. The internal reliability for these sub-scales was good with a coefficient alpha of .76 for chance and .77 for internal. Each sub-scale can range between 1 (lowest need) and 6 (highest need).

Data Analysis

The data were analyzed using STATA 11.0 (Stata Corp, College Station, TX.). The following statistical tests were used in this analysis: chi-square; ANOVA; and multinominal logistic regression. Regarding missing data, some respondents did not respond to every question, as such, some items were tabulated with less than the total number of respondents. The list-wise removal of missing data was utilized because missing cases were not missing at random (MAR).

RESULTS

Sample Characteristics

As expected, the vast majority of the respondents, 96.5 % ($n = 357$) are women. Age ranged from 20 to over 67, with approximately a third under 35 ($n = 97$, 26%), a third between the ages of 36–45 ($n = 100$, 27%), and the last third 46 years of age or older ($n = 123$, 33%). The majority of respondents are women of color with 40% ($n = 144$) identifying themselves as African American and 38% ($n = 135$) as Hispanic. The large majority of the group is either unemployed (19.4%) or receiving disability due to SLE (44%). Most of the respondents (70.4%) were diagnosed with SLE more than 5 years ago and in the last twelve months, just more than a third (37.3%, $n = 139$) were hospitalized because of complications from SLE. Respondents' most frequent type of medical coverage was Medicaid (44.7%, $n = 168$) followed by private coverage (29.1%). The majority of respondents' primary source of medical care is provided by a private physician (53.95%, $n = 191$) followed by clinics (37.9%, $n = 134$). Further demographic and socioeconomic data is listed in Table 1. The sociodemographic variables of this sample are representative of the national profile of this population regarding age, race, and ethnicity (Urowitz, Albanez, & all SLICC members, 2005).

TABLE 1 Demographics

	n	%
Gender		
Male	13	3.5
Female	357	96.5
Race		
Hispanic	135	37.7
African American	144	40.2
Asian	17	4.7
White	62	17.3
Age		
Under 21	12	3.2
21–35	97	26.1
36–45	100	26.9
46–60	123	33.1
61 and over	40	10.8
Education level		
High school or less	102	27.4
Some college	126	33.9
College graduate	108	29.0
Advanced degree	36	9.7
Employment	44	12.2
Part time		
Full time	88	24.4
Unemployed	70	19.4
On disability	159	44.0
Insurance		
Medicaid	155	44.7
Medicare	62	17.9
Private insurance	101	29.1
None	29	8.4
Admitted to hospital in past year		
Yes	121	37.3
No	203	62.7
Within year	24	6.6

SLENQ Findings

PSYCHOSOCIAL NEEDS

Each of the subscales: *Depression, Anxiety*, and *Social Economic Coping* range from 1 (no need) to 5 (high need). The scales had the following overall means: Depression 3.5 ± 1.3; anxiety 3.3 ± 1.2; and social economic coping 2.9 ± 1.3. The means indicate that respondents had the most difficulty coping with depression followed by anxiety and social economic coping. *Depression* was assessed using these items: (a) feeling depressed due to limitations caused by SLE; (b) feeling depressed because of changes in my body and; (c) feeling depressed because of side effects. *Anxiety* was assessed using the following six items: (a) feeling confused about why this disease happened to you; (b) feeling angry about having SLE; (c) feeling uncertain about the future; (d) dealing with anxiety about SLE; (e) anxiety about side effects; and (f) changes in appearance. *Social economic coping* was assessed using the following 3 items: (a) concerns about gaining employment, (b) satisfactory performance in job, and (c) coping with extra costs. The scales had the following overall means: depression, 3.5 (SD = 1.3); anxiety, 3.3 (SD = 1.2); and social economic coping, 2.9 (SD = 1.3). Reliability of the subscales was high with coefficient alphas of .91 for depression, .90 for anxiety, and .76 for economic coping.

Respondents reporting chronic symptoms or frequent flares were more likely to have higher psychosocial needs with their depression, anxiety and social economic coping as compared to those with infrequent flares. Those who reported frequent flares had a mean of 3.8 ± 1.1 for depression (p = .000); a mean of 3.7 ± 1.1 for anxiety (p = .000); and a mean of 3.3 ± 1.2 (p = .043). Respondents reporting chronic symptoms also reported significantly higher psychosocial need on depression and anxiety compared to those reporting infrequent symptoms. The means were 3.6 ± 1.2 and 3.4 ± 1.2, respectively. This reveals an association between chronic symptoms and the likelihood of higher reports of depression and anxiety, as seen in Figure 1 which displays the medians for each of these items.

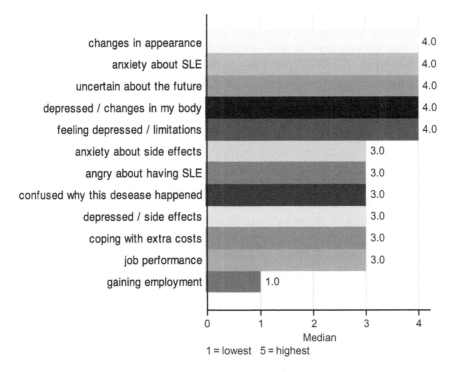

FIGURE 1 Psychosocial problems.

LOCUS OF CONTROL FINDINGS

The Multidimensional Health Locus of Control analysis demonstrated additional factors in the relationship between beliefs, perceptions and lupus disease activity (Wallston, 2010). Respondents who reported their SLE as having mostly infrequent flare-ups perceived they had more control over their health compared to those with chronic symptoms or infrequent flare-ups ($f = 6.3\, p = .002$). The chance sub-scale was not influenced by how respondents reported their experiences with SLE. Conversely, the more respondents perceived they had some control over the illness, the less likely they were to report high levels of depression or anxiety. The mean median score for chance and internal sub-scales on the Multidimensional Health Locus of Control Scale were mean 2.84 ± 1.2; median $= 2.7$ iqr $= 1.5$ and 2.98 ± 1.2; median $= 3.0$ iqr $= 1.6$, respectfully across all patients. Respondents who reported their SLE as having mostly infrequent flares (mean $= 2.5 \pm 1.2$) perceived that they had more control over their health compared to those with chronic symptoms (mean $= 2.9 \pm 1.2$) or infrequent flares (mean $= 2.8 \pm .98$) ($p = .002$).

Multinomial Analysis

Multinomial logistic regression was utilized to examine if the three psychosocial factors and locus of control influences a patient's perception of having chronic or frequent flare-ups. This method provides the relative risk ratio of the occurrence or non-occurrence of an outcome (chronic or frequent flare-ups) to a base outcome (infrequent flare-ups) by the influence of predictor variables (covariates). The rationale for using this technique was to develop a profile of patients most at risk of flare-ups.

The results of the multinomial logistic regression are presented in Table 2. The overall model was statistically significant ($X^2 = 33.9, p < .0001$). The first part of the table compares the risk of a respondent's perception of having chronic flare-ups to infrequent ones. The second portion compares the risk of a respondent's perception of having frequent flares to infrequent ones. The column labeled "rrr" in Table 1 indicates the degree to which a covariate increases or decreases the likelihood a subject will perceive having chronic or frequent flare-ups compared to infrequent ones. An rrr of 1 indicates even odds or no difference. For the "chronic model," the risk of having the perception of chronic flare-ups decreases 30% for every unit increase in locus of control ($p < .01$). The risk of perceiving chronic flare-ups increases by 60% for every unit increase in depression ($p < .01$).

Figure 2 displays that the marginal effect is statistically significant between all values of locus of control depression. The marginal effects also display the degree of increase in probability of perceiving having chronic flare-ups for a one-unit change in locus of control and depression. For the

TABLE 2 Multinomial Logistic Regression for Psychosocial Functioning

	RRR	z	P	95% CI
Chronic symptoms				
Internal	0.70	−2.55	0.01	0.53 to 0.92
Depression	1.18	2.51	0.01	1.10 to 2.32
Anxiety	0.97	−0.14	0.88	0.64 to 1.45
Social economic coping	1.08	0.64	0.56	0.83 to 1.41
Constant	1.56	0.67	0.54	0.41 to 5.82
Frequent symptoms				
Internal	0.64	−2.53	0.01	0.45 to 0.90
Depression	1.42	1.40	0.16	0.86 to 2.33
Anxiety	1.30	0.99	0.32	0.77 to 2.19
Social economic coping	1.17	0.96	0.33	0.84 to 1.64
Constant	0.26	−1.46	0.14	0.04 to 1.56

Base comparison = infrequent flare-ups.

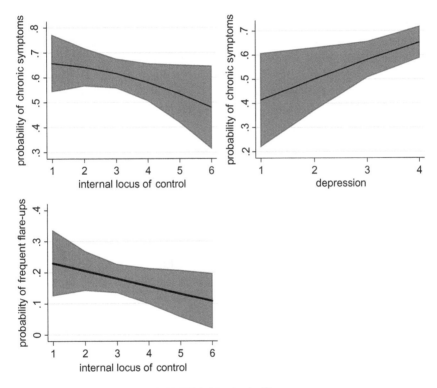

FIGURE 2 Marginal effects.

"frequent flare-up model," the risk of having the perception of frequent flare-ups decreases 60% for every unit increase in locus of control ($p < .01$).

Figure 2 displays that the marginal effect is statistically significant between all values of locus of control and depression. The marginal effects also display the degree of increase in probability of perceiving having chronic flare-ups for a one-unit change in locus of control and depression. As locus of control increases from 1 to 6, the probability of having the perception of chronic flare-ups decreases from 66% to 48% ($p < .01$). As depression increases from 1 to 4, the probability of having the perception of "chronic flare-ups" increases from 41% to 65%. Finally, as locus of control increases from 1 to 6, the probability of "frequent flare-ups" decreases from 23% to 11%.

DISCUSSION

As the findings indicate, locus of control and depression significantly influence the degree to which patients are likely to perceive chronic or frequent flare-ups. Therefore, patient beliefs about their ability to control lupus are a key component in how they experience the chronicity and the acuity of the illness. Learning that depression and locus of control can influence a patients' perception of disease activity is important because the more control patients feel they have, the less depressed they may be and less chronic their symptoms appear. This is an important dimension for mental health providers to understand because stress is both a trigger and response to SLE and effectively managing stress is a key goal of psychosocial intervention (Braden, McGlone, & Pennington, 1993; Jolly & Utset, 2004; Jolly, 2005; Karlson, Liang, & Eaton, 2004).

We see from this study's findings that feelings such as depression and perceptions of one's illness may distort or prolong the feeling of being ill. While depression is part of the relationship between locus of control and disease activity, anxiety did not present as part of this equation. This is different from other studies (DiMatteo et al., 2000; Greco, Rudy, & Manzi, 2004). There is emerging evidence that CBT interventions can interrupt and moderate the cycle of disease activity-negative perceptions-disease activity (Ng Petrus-Chan, 2007). The more we are able to identify these potential patterns, the better able we may be to assist patients to cope adaptively by enhancing their sense of control over lupus and modifying their negative emotional states (Haupt et al., 2005). If interventions are effective in this task, the patient will be more likely to: (a) report symptoms more accurately and (b) manage their emotional reactions, which can be emotionally and physically harmful for the lupus patient. In this way, the recursive cycle of negative emotional state, disease activity and resulting negative emotional state may be re-aligned to a more adaptive relationship.

Lupus patients would benefit from a multimodal approach that emphasizes biopsychosocial framework, which addresses the physical realities of lupus activity as well as the social, psychological and emotional aspects of the illness. During a flare, lupus patients would be particularly aided by relaxation techniques, deep breathing, mental imagery, progressive muscle relaxation, and biofeedback. These self-management interventions should be a central component of care for lupus patients who are experiencing intermittent or regular flares of the illness.

Alongside a biopsychosocial approach, a reliance on CBT has emerged as a useful approach in helping lupus patients identify their thought and behavior patterns and manage their illness with more mindfulness (Greco et al., 2004; Sohng, 2003). CBT with lupus patients has shown that those who have participated in SBT trainings have shown less depression and less fatigue than others who received no interventions (Sohng, 2003). Regarding stress-reduction in lupus patients, CBT-based stress-reduction program, participants had significantly greater reductions in pain and psychological dysfunctions compared with the usual medical care group (Greco et al., 2004). As Navarrete-Navarrete et al. (2002) concur, patients who received CBT show "improved level of physical functioning, vitality, general health perceptions and mental health, compared with the group of patients who only received conventional care" (Navarrete-Navarrete et al., 2002, p. 169). CBT can help patients attend to what they think and say about their illness and provide a method of redirecting their thinking in a positive direction. Furthermore, clients can be helped to recognize their self-talk attitudes and identify beliefs that make it more difficult for them to live with this chronic condition (Digeronimo, 2002).

CONCLUSION

Whether the health care provider is the treating physician, nurse, social worker, or any other member of a health care team, it is essential to assess this population for how their beliefs and perceptions may impact the disease activity, their self-care, their medication compliance, and so on. The evidence from this study and related literature indicate the efficacy of CBT alongside other bio-psycho-social interventions to enhance patients' ability to cope with this chronic autoimmune illness (Greco, Rudy, & Manzi, 2004; Sohng, 2003).

Future research should attempt to further clarify what types of interventions within CBT are the most effective in assisting patients to moderate their negative emotional states. Another area of future research should address the culturally influenced perceptions of health and illness as this is an essential component to assessment and counseling for patients with lupus. Additionally, as lupus disproportionately affects women, it would be critical to explore how the role of gender influences the experience of chronic illness and health care. Findings from this study have underscored the importance of continued research on the psychosocial impact of chronic disease processes, with an emphasis on how patients' beliefs often impact physical and mental health outcomes.

REFERENCES

Babul, J.E., Calderon, J., Gonzalez, M., Martinez, M.E. Bravo-Zehnder, M., Henriquez, C., Jacobelli, S., Gonzalez, A., & Massardo, L. (2011). Common mental disorders and psychological distress in systemic lupus erythematosus are not associated with disease activity. *Lupus, 20*(1), 58–66.

Bachen, E.A, Chesney, M.A, & Criswell, L.A. (2009). Prevalence of mood and anxiety disorders in women with systemic lupus erythematosus. *Arthritis Rheumatology, 61*(6), 822–829.

Beckerman, N.L., Auerbach, C., & Blanco, I. (2011). Psychosocial dimensions of SLE: Implications for the health care team. *Multidisciplinary Journal of Health Care, 4*(4), 67–72.

Bertoli, A.M, Vila, L.M., Apte, M., Fessler, B.J., Bastian, H.M., Reveille, J.D., and Alcarcon, G.S. (2007). Systemic Lupus Erythematosus in a multiethnic US Cohort LUMINA XLVII: Factors predictive of pulmonary damage. *Lupus, 16*(6), 410–417.

Braden, C.J., McGlone, K., & Pennington, F. (1993). Specific psychosocial and behavioral outcomes from the systemic lupus erythematosus self-help-course. *Health Education Quarterly, 20*, 29–41.

Carr, F.N., Nicassion, P.M., & Ishimori, M.L. (2011). Depression predicts self-reported disease activity in systemic lupus erythematosus. *Lupus, 20*(1), 80–84.

Daleboudt, G.M., Broadbent, E., Berger, S.P., & Kaptein, A.A. (2011). Illness perceptions in patients with systemic lupus erythematosus and proliferative lupus nephritis *Lupus, 20*, 290–298.

Danoff-Burg, S., & Friedberg, F. (2009). Unmet needs of patients with SLE. *Behavioral Medicine, 35*(1), 5–14.

Digeronimo, T.F. (2002). *New hope for people with lupus*. Roseville, CA: Prima Publishing.

DiMatteo, M.R., Lepper, H.S., & Croghan, T.W. (2000). Depression is a risk factor for noncompliance with medical treatment: Meta-analysis of the effects of anxiety and depression on patient adherence. *Archives of Internal Medicine, 160*, 2101–2107.

Dobkin, P.L., DaCosta, D., & Fortin, P.R. (2001). Living with lupus: A prospective pan-Canadian study. *Journal of Rheumatology, 28*, 2442–2448.

Dobkin, P., Fortin, P.R., Joseph L, Esdaile, J.M., Danoff, D.S., & Clarke, A.E. (1998). Psychosocial contributors to mental and physical health in patients with SLE. *Arthritis Care Research, 11*, 23–31.

Duvdevany, M., Cohen, A., Minsker-Valtzer, A., & Lorber, M. (2011). Psychological correlates of adherence to self-care, disease activity and functioning in persons with systemic lupus erythematosus. *Lupus, 20*, 14–22.

Giffords, E.D. (2003). Understanding and managing systemic lupus erythematosus (SLE). *Social Work in Health Care, 37*, 57–72.

Gladman, D.D., Urowitz, M.B., Ong, A., Gough, J., & MacKinnon A. (1996). Lack of correlation among the 3 outcomes describing SLE: Disease activity, damage and quality of life. *Clinical Experimental Rheumatology, 14*, 305–308.

Goodman, D., Morrissey, S., & Graham, D. (2005). Illness representations of SLE. *Qualitative Health, 15*(5), 606–619.

Greco, C.M., Rudy, T.H., & Manzi, S. (2004). Effects of a stress-reduction program on psychological function, pain and physical function of systemic lupus erythematosus patients: a randomized controlled trial. *Arthritis and Rheumatology*, *51*, 625–634.

Grotz, M., Hapke, U., Lampert, T., & Baumeister, H. (2011). Health locus of control and health behavior: Results from a nationally representative survey. *Psychology in Health Medicine*, *16*(2), 129–140.

Haupt, M., Millen, S., Jänner, M., Falagan, D., Fischer-Betz, R., & Schneider, M. (2005). Improvement of coping abilities in patients with systemic lupus erythematosus: A prospective study. *Annals of Rheumatologic Diseases*, *64*(11), 1618–1623.

Iverson, G. (2002). Screening for depression in systemic lupus erythematosus with the British Columbia Major Depression. *Psychological Research*, *90*, 1091–1096.

Jolly, M. (2005). How does quality of life of patients with systemic lupus erythematosus compare with that of other common chronic illnesses? *Journal of Rheumatology*, 32, 1706–1718.

Jolly, M., & Utset, T.O. (2004). Can disease specific measures for systemic lupus erythematosus predict patients' health related quality of life. *Lupus*, *13*, 924–926.

Karlson, E.W., Liang, M.H., & Eaton, H. (2004). A randomized clinical trial of a psychoeducational intervention to improve outcomes in systemic lupus erythematosus. *Arthritis Rheumatology*, *50*, 1832–1841.

Khanna, S.H., Pandey, R.M., & Handa, R. (2004). The relationship between disease activity and quality of life in systemic lupus erythematosus. *Rheumatology*, *43*(12), 1536–1540.

Kozora, E., Ellison, M.C., Waxmonsky, J.A, Wamboldt, F.S, & Patterson, T.L. (2005). Major life stress, coping styles, and social support in relation to psychological distress in patients with systemic lupus erythematosus. *Lupus*, *14*, 363–372.

Kulczycka, L., Sysa-Jedrzejowska, A., & Robak, E. (2010). Quality of life and satisfaction with life in SLE patients-the importance of clinical manifestations. *Clinical Rheumatology*, *29*(9), 991–997.

Kuriya, B., Gladman, D.D., Ibañez, D., & Urowitz, M.B. (2008). Quality of life over time in patients with systemic lupus erythematosus. *Arthritis Care Research*, *59*, 181–185.

Lindner, H., & Lederman, L. (2009). Relationship of illness perceptions with depression among individuals diagnosed with lupus. *Depression & Anxiety*, *26*(6), 575–582.

McElhone, K., Abbott, J., Gray, J., Williams, A., Teh, L.-S. (2010). Patient perspective of systemic lupus erythematosus in relation to health-related quality of life concepts: A qualitative study. *Lupus*, *19*(14), 1640–1647.

McElhone, K., Abbott, J., & Teh, L.S. (2009). A review of health related quality of life in systemic lupus erythematosus. *Lupus*, *15*(10), 633–643.

Monaghan, S.M., Sharpe, L., Denton, F., Levy, J., Schreiber, L., & Sensky, T. (2007). Relationship between appearance and psychological distress in rheumatic diseases. *Arthritis Rheumatology*, *57*(2), 303–309.

Moses, N., Wiggers, J., Nicholas, C., & Cockburn, J. (2005). Prevalence and correlates of perceived unmet needs of people with systemic lupus erythematosus. *Patient Education Counseling*, *57*(1), 30–38.

Navarrete-Navarrete, N., Peralta-Ramírez, M.I., Sabio-Sánchez, J.M., Coín, M.A., Robles-Ortega, H., Hidalgo-Tenorio, C., . . . Jiménez-Alonso, J. (2002). Efficacy of cognitive behavioural therapy for the treatment of chronic stress in patients with lupus erythematosus: A randomized controlled trial. *Psychotherapy and Psychosomatics, 79*(2), 163-179.

Nery, F.G., Borba, E.F., Hatch, J.P., Soares, E.-J.C., Bonfa, E., & Neto, F.L. (2007). Major depressive disorder and disease activity in systemic lupus erythematosus. *Comprehensive Psychiatry, 48,* 14–19.

Ng Petrus-Chan, W. (2007). Group psychosocial program for enhancing psycho-logical well-being of people with systemic lupus erythematosus. *Lupus, 6*(3), 75–87.

Nowicka-Sauer, K. (2007). Patients' perspective: Lupus in patients' drawings. *Clinical Rheumatology, 26*(9), 1523–1525.

Pereira, L.S., Araújo, L.G., Sampaio, R.F., & Haddad, J.P. (2011). Factorial analysis of the Multidimensional Health Locus of Control Scale—Form C for elderly. *Revista Brasileira de Fisioterapia, 15*(5), 363–370.

Pierce, A. (2008). Uncovering the mysteries of immunity, and of lupus. *The New York Times*, A, 11.

Pons-Estel, G.J., Alarcon, G.S., Scofield, L., Reinlib, L., & Cooper, G.S. (2010). Understanding the epidemiology and progression of systemic lupus erythematosus. *Seminars in Arthritis and Rheumatism, 39*(4), 257–273.

Rahman, A., & Isenberg, D.A. (2008). Systemic Lupus Erythematosus. *New England Journal of Medicine, 358*(9), 929–939.

Robles, T.F., Glaser, R., & Kiecolt-Glaser, J.K. (2005). Out of balance: A new look at chronic stress, depression, and immunity. *Current Directions in Psychological Science, 14,* 111–115.

Seawell, A.H., & Danoff-Burg, S. (2004). Psychosocial research on SLE: A literature review. *Lupus, 13*(12), 891–899.

Seguí, J., Ramos-Casals, M., García-Carrasco, M., de Flores, T., Cervera, R., Valdés, M., Font, J., & Ingelmo, M. (2000). Psychiatric and psychosocial disorders in patients with systemic lupus erythematosus: A longitudinal study of active and inactive stages of the disease. *Lupus, 9,* 584–588.

Shorthall, E., Isenberg, D., & Newman, S. (1995). Factors associated with mood and mood disorders in SLE Lupus. *Lupus, 4,* 272–279.

Sohng, K.Y. (2003). Effects of a self-management course for patients with systemic lupus erythematosus. *Journal of Advanced Nursing, 42,* 479–486.

Stevens, N.R., Hamilton, N.A., & Wallston, K.A. (2011). Validation of the MHLOC scales for labor and delivery. *Research in Nursing Health, 34*(4), 282–296.

Urowitz, M.B., Albanez, D., & all SLICC members. (2005). Systemic Lupus International Collaborating Clinics (SLICC) Inception Cohort Registry to study risk factors for atherosclerosis: Initial report [abstract]. *Arthritis Rheum, 50*(Suppl 9), S594–S595.

Wallace, D.J. (2000). *The lupus book*. New York, NY: Oxford University Press.

Wallston, K.A. (2010). Validity of the multidimensional health locus of control scales in American sign language. *Journal of Health Psychology, 15,* 1064–1074.

Wallston, B.S., & DeVellis, R.F. (1978). Development of the multidimensional health locus of control (MHLC) scales. *Health Education Monographs, 6,* 160–170.

Wang, C., Mayo, N.E., & Fortin, P.R. (2001). The relationship between health related quality of life and disease activity and damage in Systemic Lupus Erythematosus. *Journal of Rheumatology, 28,* 525–532.

Lupus and Community-Based Social Work

WENDY SCHUDRICH, MSW
*Wurzweiler School of Social Work, Yeshiva University, New York,
New York, USA*

DIANE GROSS, MPH and JESSICA ROWSHANDEL, MSW
S.L.E. Lupus Foundation, New York, New York, USA

*Systemic lupus erythematous (SLE) is a chronic autoimmune
disease that disproportionately strikes women of color. SLE patients
frequently experience physical, emotional, and social challenges
that often result in unmet biopsychosocial needs. Because of the
nature of the disease and the needs of patients, agencies serving SLE patients that engage in community-based social work can
positively impact their clients' lives. The S.L.E. Lupus Foundation
participates in a myriad of community-based social work practices
to help address the needs of their clients. These services include
helping economically disadvantaged patients access appropriate
services within their communities, building awareness about SLE
in society, connecting with government officials at all levels, and
collaborating with health care organizations to serve those affected
by SLE. Specific examples of community-based activities at the
S.L.E. Lupus Foundation are described in detail.*

INTRODUCTION

An estimated 1.5 million Americans suffer from systemic lupus erythematous
(SLE), a chronic autoimmune disease. Approximately 90% of SLE, or lupus,
patients are women (Wallace, 2008), and SLE disproportionately affects

Black, Hispanic, First Nation and Asian women (Alarcón et al., 2004). Black and Asian women are two to three times more likely to develop the disease, for example, than White women (S.L.E. Lupus Foundation, n.d.). People of color are more likely to develop more severe manifestations of the disease, more severe disease activity and overall damage and higher mortality rates (Moses, Wiggers, Nicholas, & Cockburn, 2005; Pons-Estel, Alarcón, Scofield, Reinlib, & Cooper, 2010).

Chronic Illness and Biopsychosocial Needs

People with any chronic illness often deal with similar physical, emotional, and social challenges that result in common biopsychosocial needs. Biopsychosocial difficulties often center on the patient's ability to address the demands of his or her illness while simultaneously trying to achieve a fulfilling, independent life (Whittemore & Dixon, 2008).

Upon diagnosis, people with chronic illnesses frequently experience troubling emotional responses including depression, anxiety, fear, anger, and apathy (Whittemore & Dixon, 2008). While this may be the beginning of a patient's challenges, Whittemore and Dixon (2008) explain that, as disease courses change over time, biopsychosocial needs can also change over time. For example, coping strategies that may be functional for a patient at one point in his or her illness may not be sufficient at other points, and patients need to develop new ways of managing. "Ongoing resources and support appear to be critical factors in providing assistance" to patients with chronic illnesses (Whittemore & Dixon, 2008, p. 185).

Critical resources for helping patients with chronic illnesses to navigate challenges associated with disease include family, friends, support groups, and counselors. The range of help that patients receive includes physical assistance with day-to-day activities, emotional support, and companionship (Whittemore & Dixon, 2008). Therefore, Whittemore and Dixon (2008) recommend a multidisciplinary approach to addressing patients' social, emotional, physical, and vocational needs. Finally, there is some evidence to suggest that emotional states can have an impact on the physical manifestations of chronic illnesses in addition to illnesses effecting emotional distress. (Beckerman, Auerbach, & Blanco, 2011; Treharne, Kitas, Lyons, & Booth, 2005). This, then, would suggest great benefit to understanding and addressing both the physical and psychosocial needs of patients with chronic illnesses.

Biopsychosocial Needs of Individuals With Lupus

Studies of lupus patients indicate that these individuals have similar biopsychosocial needs as people with other chronic illnesses although lupus patients have some additional needs that are unique to their condition

(Alarcón et al., 2004; Jump et al., 2005; Kozora, Ellison, Waxmonsky, Wamboldt, & Patterson, 2005). Lupus can be an invisible illness that adds another layer of complication because those afflicted with these conditions often lack obvious visible manifestations of disease. Patients may experience suspicion and withdrawal by others in addition to experiencing the physical, emotional, and other psychosocial challenges associated with their disease (Donoghue & Siegel, 2000). As a result, patients with invisible chronic illnesses can experience "shame and insecurity that can generate a vicious cycle of insecurity, depression, and social isolation" (Greenhalgh, 2009, p. 631). This can result in a lack of physical assistance with day-to-day activities and emotional support when it is most needed.

As lupus disproportionally affects people of color, some recent studies have examined the needs of minority lupus patients compared to White patients. Black and Latina patients have greater unmet physical, emotional, and socioeconomic needs than their White counterparts (Beckerman et al., 2011; Danoff-Burg & Friedberg, 2009). Additionally, Black SLE patients report more severe manifestations of lupus and more physical problems with their illness than White patients, including more difficulty managing symptoms of tiredness, not sleeping well, pain, and feeling worse after physical activity (Danoff-Burg et al., 2009; Fernández et al., 2007).

Unmet financial needs of lupus patients have been identified in several studies. These include needing help managing costs related to SLE, meeting basic living expenses, and managing employment because of problems related to lupus (Beckerman et al., 2011; Danoff-Burg & Friedberg, 2009). Lupus tends to impact people in their prime earning years, and many patients rely on public assistance. Chronic diseases with early onset have a negative impact on earnings and the ability to accrue for retirement (Yelin et al., 2007). A study of people employed at the time of lupus diagnosis found that by 5 years after diagnosis, 15% had stopped working, by 10 years, 36% had stopped working, and by 15 years, 51% had stopped working. On average, these individuals were diagnosed in their mid-thirties; therefore, almost none were employed to a typical retirement age (Yelin et al., 2007). A study of employment and work disability for people with lupus found that 33% of patients were on work disability while 47% were employed. Work disability was related to "a variety of psychosocial and disease related factors, including age, race, sex, SES [socioeconomic status], education, disease activity and duration, pain, fatigue, anxiety, and neurocognitive involvement" (Baker & Pope, 2009, p. 284).

Moses and colleagues (2005) have noted that, due to numerous unmet physical, daily living, and psychological needs, current health care services are not adequate for some people with lupus. Additionally, "referrals to organizations that provide support and information to persons with chronic illness are an important supplement to the medical treatment of SLE" (Danoff-Burg & Friedberg, 2009, p. 12).

Community Social Work and Lupus

Community social work is macro-practice. That is, using social work skills usually associated with direct individual or group practice (e.g., engagement), community social workers seek to assist larger groups of people with some common characteristics that come together to form a community (Hardcastle, Powers, & Wenocur, 2011). Community social workers typically engage in advocacy, social action, and community organizing (Hardcastle et al., 2011; Hepworth, Rooney, Rooney, Strom-Gottfried, & Larsen, 2009). They engage directly with members of the defined community and community partners, facilitate collaboration with other organizations, disseminate public information, network, engage in social marketing, and share information with the public (Hardcastle et al., 2011; Hepworth et al., 2009). Frequently, social workers will simultaneously engage in both macro-practice and direct practice with either individual clients or smaller groups (Hardcastle et al., 2011).

Lupus, in particular, is an appropriate practice area for agencies and practitioners engaged in community social work as they have a high level of unmet psychosocial needs. Since lupus is difficult to diagnose, community-based social work activities can be used to inform the public about the disease in order to help patients identify themselves. This may be of particular assistance in communities of color with higher incidences of lupus so that psychoeducation and social support networks are prominently available. Finally, community-based social work can help engage clients and serve as a gateway to services for lupus patients with unmet physical, psychological, emotional, or socioeconomic needs. Community-based social work in the lupus community draws on the whole systems approach and the critical health approach in the prevention and management of chronic illness (Greenhalgh, 2009).

One way to better understand how community-based social work can positively impact patients with lupus is to examine an organization doing this work more closely. The S.L.E. Lupus Foundation of New York is one such organization.

THE S.L.E. LUPUS FOUNDATION

The S.L.E. Lupus Foundation ("Foundation") is a New York City-based organization whose mission is to provide direct services, education, public awareness, and funding for lupus research. They aim to address racial disparities through community-based outreach programs serving minority populations and effective advocacy at national, state, and local levels. The Foundation is headquartered in New York City and also has a West Coast division in Los Angeles. While the Foundation has offices in three boroughs (Bronx, Brooklyn, and Manhattan), it has a presence throughout all five boroughs (Bronx, Brooklyn, Manhattan [Midtown and Upper Manhattan], Staten Island, and Queens). Additionally, the Foundation regularly collaborates with other lupus organizations throughout the state and nationally in order to serve clients. All services to clients are provided free-of-charge.

Biopsychosocial Needs of the Foundation's Clients

One of the most common presenting problems for the Foundation's clients is lack of social or emotional support. New clients frequently report that family or friends do not understand the actual experiences of patients with lupus. For example, a client experiencing extreme fatigue may be told by well-meaning family to "just get out of bed" or to "try a little harder." Another problem for Foundation clients is the loss of friendships or other social connections since lupus patients may not have the energy to engage in social activities that they previously enjoyed. A study of the Foundation's membership that looked at the unique psychosocial challenges of this group, found that survey respondents had the most difficulty coping with depression, followed by anxiety and socioeconomic coping and that the greater the perceived sense of control over their condition, the less likely they were to report feeling depressed and anxious (Beckerman et al., 2011).

Other problems for Foundation clients include the financial ramifications of having a chronic illness that limits an individual's ability to work. Because of temporary employment interruptions or job loss, patients seek Foundation financial assistance to help meet basic needs critical for their well-being, such as medication, rent, or utilities. Another common example of financial need is that clients may need assistance purchasing clothing due to weight fluctuations from steroid use, which can increase a patient's weight temporarily, but rapidly.

Services Offered by the S.L.E. Lupus Foundation

Lupus has a significant impact on quality of life due to the physical and psychological aspects of the disease and the economic burden of medical costs and job reduction or loss. The S.L.E. Lupus Foundation has programs that reach thousands of people every year to address these needs. From educational workshops with renowned medical professionals to one-on-one counseling sessions with the Foundation's staff social worker. The Programs & Social Services Team is constantly assessing their members' needs to ensure they are offering services that meet clients' varied requirements.

The Foundation's Programs and Social Services Team is comprised of a National Director of Program Development, a Director of Social Services, both of whom work out of the Midtown Manhattan headquarters, and two bilingual Outreach Coordinators who staff the Lupus Cooperative of New York offices in the Bronx and Brooklyn.

The Lupus Cooperative of New York (LCNY) is a decade-old grassroots, community-based effort that helps economically disadvantaged people living with lupus access quality health care, social services, and financial resources. They also aim to facilitate timely diagnosis and treatment. The program has an integrated network of community partnerships including community health providers, social service organizations and local businesses to improve health outcomes for those living with lupus. Outreach centers located in the Bronx and Brooklyn are each staffed by a bilingual outreach coordinator. Due to financial constraints, the presence of a full time coordinator in Northern Manhattan was scaled back to a partnership with a local health center to provide essential educational, outreach, and referral services in that community. The Foundation is working to reinstate a full time presence in Northern Manhattan by the end of 2012. In patients with a chronic disease, such as lupus, social support has been shown to act "as a protective factor or buffer, making it possible for patients and their families to navigate the health and social systems, utilize them, and benefit from them" (Pons-Estel et al., 2010, p. 263). This is the focus of the LCNY, which assists low-income, disadvantaged, individuals with lupus and their families.

In addition to these outreach centers, the Director of Social Services provides additional services to clients throughout New York City, including one-on-one counseling, support groups in addition to those at LCNY, and an online monthly advice column that covers psychosocial topics such as coping with lupus, travel, and work issues.

The Programs and Social Services Team, as a whole, assists individuals with lupus through direct support services that include help resolving difficulties related to health care, housing, employment, personal finances, education and emotional issues. Specific services include bilingual and monolingual peer-guided ongoing support groups, physician and other health care referrals, one-on-one counseling, emergency grants, nutrition and exercise workshops, referrals regarding social services and benefits and assistance filling out applications, education sessions for other community-based agencies, provider education, participation in health fairs, monthly advice column, and bilingual health education materials.

Community Social Work at the S.L.E. Lupus Foundation

Community social work at the Foundation focuses on numerous activities with the goal of reaching and connecting different segments of the lupus community and building awareness about relevant issues in the broader society. The Foundation connects with government officials at the city, state, and national levels. The Foundation engages in community-based activities in order to reach out to patients who are already diagnosed with lupus and to build awareness about lupus in order to help patients who may not yet be diagnosed connect to appropriate services. Furthermore, the Foundation works with health care providers through several venues in order to help them better understand lupus and issues related to the illness so that they may better serve their patients. Finally, the Foundation collaborates with a host of other organizations whose services are often needed by SLE patients.

THE S.L.E. LUPUS FOUNDATION AND GOVERNMENTAL COMMUNITY SOCIAL WORK

At least once a year, Foundation staff meet with New York City Council members. The goal of these meetings is, at times, to secure funding, but it is also to build a broader awareness about lupus. Council Members are regularly updated on Foundation activities and issues important to lupus patients. The Foundation activities in this area are particularly important as they relate to building awareness in public servants whose constituents may be made up of cultural groups who are traditionally underserved by the medical community and who are at greater risk for developing lupus.

On a statewide level, the Foundation partners with other organizations as part of the Lupus Agencies of New York State (LANYS). LANYS works on building awareness and engaging in advocacy to assist the larger lupus community in New York State. Previous efforts at this level have included an annual exhibit on lupus at the New York State Fair, initiating legislation to designate May as Lupus Awareness Month in New York State, and advocating for policies protecting lupus patients' access to affordable drugs. LANYS is currently promoting two bills in the state legislature to help support those with lupus.

On the national level, the Foundation is part of the Lupus Research Institute (LRI) National Coalition. The Coalition is a group of lupus patient services and advocacy organizations located in major urban markets across the country. The Coalition works to ensure funds for lupus research, protect the rights of people with lupus to get and keep adequate health care insurance coverage, eliminate racial disparities, promote education and awareness of the seriousness of lupus, and empower people to effectively advocate for themselves for improved treatments and a cure.

For example, the Coalition successfully petitioned for Congressional funding for a national lupus health education program for physicians and health care providers. The Lupus Initiative, funded by the federal Offices of Minority Health, Women's Health and Surgeon General, is aimed at alleviating racial disparities by providing health care professionals with state-of-the-art training to recognize, diagnose, and treat lupus appropriately. This innovative program includes enhanced medical education curriculum and continuing medical education credits aimed at reducing the impact of health disparities in the diagnosis and care management of people with lupus.

COMMUNITY SOCIAL WORK AT THE S.L.E. LUPUS FOUNDATION:
REACHING OUT TO PATIENTS

The Foundation recognizes the numerous unmet biopsychosocial needs of individuals with lupus, including those who may be undiagnosed (Beckerman et al., 2011; Danoff-Burg & Friedberg, 2009; Jump et al., 2005; Kozora et al., 2005). In order to reach these patients, the Foundation engages in a wide array of outreach activities that include collaborating with other health organizations, providing information at health fairs, and public awareness campaigns.

The LCNY outreach model is specifically designed to help address racial disparities and access to health care for people of color with lupus. Through LCNY, the Foundation staffs two bilingual outreach coordinators who go into neighborhoods comprised of traditionally underserved populations to help identify community members who have or may have lupus. Once contact is made with patients, other social work services that the Foundation offers are made available within the community to help address the most pressing unmet biopsychosocial needs for individuals with lupus, discussed above.

The Foundation found that it is important to reach people through conventional and unconventional methods. Their bilingual lupus education brochures are distributed in settings that attract young, women of color who are candidates for lupus. These include places such as beauty salons, places of worship, community centers, daycare centers, *bodegas*, schools, and more. More formal methods of outreach are done also, such as attending health fairs within a variety of New York City communities, as well as educating staff from other community-based agencies about lupus. This is particularly relevant if these community-based agencies are located within communities of color and underprivileged communities. With participation in health fairs, alone, the LCNY Outreach Coordinators reached over 8,500 people between January 2011 and September 2011; these numbers reinforce the need for continued participation in community-based events.

In order to expand the breadth of its outreach programs, in 2011 the Foundation launched a Corporate Outreach program. In collaboration with human resources departments, the Foundation provides presentations about lupus to groups of employees in an effort to educate employers, supervisors, and colleagues about the biopsychosocial needs of workers with lupus, and information to help people identify symptoms in themselves, colleagues, friends, and families.

REACHING PATIENTS THROUGH NEW MEDIA AND TECHNOLOGY

The Foundation has realized that online media is an important way to reach underserved communities beyond New York City. In 2011, the Foundation started providing webinars that can be easily accessed worldwide by telephone and/or Internet. Recent webinars have covered numerous topics and have included *Tools for Managing Your Lupus, Benlysta—The FDA Approved It, But Is It Right for Me?*, and *Lupus and Pregnancy*. The talks are given by renowned rheumatologists who partner with the Foundation to provide these services to patients. Future topics will address biopsychosocial issues in addition to medical issues.

The Foundation also utilizes social networking sites like Facebook and Twitter to share information with their members and clients and to also reach a larger audience. This allows the Foundation to provide information on the latest lupus developments and on upcoming events and support groups. Furthermore, it offers a place for people to share information and learn from each other. For example, the monthly advice column written by the Director of Social Services is posted on Facebook each month in addition to the Foundation's website. It often prompts much discussion, provides the social worker with a new way to reach out to people who express a desire for services or a need, and provides an added way for patients to reach out to and support each other. A realization of the need for call-in support groups, which the social worker will pilot in 2012 and will be available to lupus patients nationally came from the Foundation's activity on Facebook.

REACHING PATIENTS THROUGH ORGANIZATIONAL COLLABORATION

The Foundation regularly collaborates with other health care organizations to sponsor or co-sponsor programs that are viewed as helpful to Foundation clients and family members. One such event is the annual *Get Into the Loop & Learn About Lupus—New York City Hospital Tour*. In this month-long program, physicians give a talk in a hospital in each of the five boroughs on a topic of interest to patients with lupus. Before the talk, dinner is provided to participants. The goal of the annual Hospital Tour is to further educate lupus patients about timely and relevant topics related to lupus and to facilitate mutual support among participants. The Hospital Tour also provides patients with access to doctors and other health care providers; they are able to ask them questions in a group setting and get their questions answered.

Another example of how the Foundation collaborates with other health care organizations is in the coordination of the annual program entitled *Living Life Healthy with Lupus*, which is co-sponsored with the Hospital for Special Surgery. This program seeks to help patients with SLE learn more about living a healthy lifestyle while enjoying a little pampering. Participants can register for complimentary services that include hairstyling, makeup application, and massages. Additionally, demonstrations on feel-good activities such as Tai Chi are also available. Lunchtime speakers share ideas about wellness that are specific to individuals with SLE.

In collaboration with the Long Island University (LIU) Department of Occupational Therapy, patients in Brooklyn were able to participate in a

Lupus Aquatics Program. The first lupus aquatics class was held for six weeks in the fall of 2009. These 6-week sessions used stretching, balance, and gentle aerobic activities to strengthen the whole body. Due to the success of this program, they offered a second aquatics class in the fall of 2010, an 8-week Tai-Chi aquatics class. This exercise helps to reduce muscle and joint pain and is ideal for creating improved range of motion and mobility. The lupus aquatics program is now in its third year. It is hoped that this class will continue to be offered annually and be expanded to be offered twice a year, in the spring and fall. In addition, an elective Lupus Aquatics course was developed and is available for LIU Sport Medicine and Health Care Students.

A chronic disease self-management class is offered once a year in collaboration with the Family Health Center at North General Hospital in Manhattan. This 6-week program meets 2 hours per week and covers topics such as coping with stress, fatigue, pain and isolation; exercise and nutrition; medication usage; and improving communication with family, friends, and health professionals. The objective of this program is to educate participants on the importance of managing their disease.

This year, a 10-week nutrition workshop, in collaboration with the Cornell University Cooperative Extension, was held in the Foundation's Manhattan office and in their Brooklyn location. One is planned at their Bronx site later this year, although this is where the program was first held 2 years ago. The NYC Expanded Food & Nutrition Education Program is a free program for low-income child caregivers to teach them how to make healthy food choices with a limited budget and how to pass this information along to the children they care for. Participants meet once a week for an interactive discussion about nutrition and meal preparation. The group was led by a Community Educator from Cornell. At the end of the 10 weeks, each participant was awarded a certificate, which Cornell University encourages them to put on their resumé. This addresses multiple needs of the lupus patient: proper nutrition for themselves and their families, especially designed for those on a limited income, and proficiency that can translate into a job skill.

The purpose of these inter-organizational relationships is, typically, to enlarge the scope of services that each organization provides. Within each partnership, more patients can be reached and more services can be offered.

REACHING OUT TO PATIENTS AND PUBLIC AWARENESS CAMPAIGNS

The Foundation always looks for opportunities and partnerships that allow them to educate the general public about lupus both locally and nationally. For the previous 3 years, during the month of October, the Foundation has been granted free space by EHE International for a 115-square foot display window in Rockefeller Plaza in order to generate awareness about lupus.

This exhibit draws attention to this often undiagnosed disease through facts and film.

In addition, the Foundation is collaborating with CBS Cares on a public service announcement (PSA) what is scheduled to launch in early 2012. CBS Cares is a campaign where talent from many CBS programs is featured in a PSA that airs on national television and is promoted on their web site.

COMMUNITY SOCIAL WORK AT THE S.L.E. LUPUS FOUNDATION: REACHING OUT TO HEALTH CARE PROVIDERS

The Foundation provides direct services to lupus patients, but it also participates in activities to assist the medical community that serves lupus patients. As a result, the Foundation engages in outreach to physicians that provide medical care to lupus patients and other medically oriented institutions, including hospitals and professional organizations.

The Foundation endeavors to develop relationships with individual physicians and practices that treat individuals with lupus. This typically includes rheumatologists, but also includes general practitioners and specialists who address complications of lupus. The purpose of developing these relationships is twofold. First, the Foundation seeks to compile a comprehensive list of physicians who are well versed in treating lupus patients so they can build a referral network for their clients. Additionally, the Foundation aims to be of assistance to physicians as well as patients.

The relationship that the Foundation develops with individual physicians and practices varies based on the needs and requests of each medical practice. In the simplest case, the Foundation will periodically provide materials about Foundation services to the practice, and the practice will make the materials available to patients. In other situations, Foundation staff will meet individually with physicians to help them begin to address some of the biopsychosocial needs of patients.

CONCLUSION

The clients served by the S.L.E. Lupus Foundation have many of the same needs as those identified in previous studies. The Foundation recognizes that needs vary due to differences in socioeconomic status, education, and the specific lupus symptoms of the patient and tailors its services to meet the various patient needs. Since communities of color are disproportionately vulnerable to lupus, the Foundation focuses many education and outreach services in underserved communities through the LCNY. As noted in earlier studies on the unmet needs of patients with SLE, emotional and social support are often the most pressing needs of clients of the Foundation (Beckerman et al., 2011; Danoff-Burg & Friedberg, 2009; Donoghue & Siegel,

2000; Greenhalgh, 2009; Moses et al., 2005; Whittemore & Dixon, 2008). Through its array of individual and group services, the Foundation seeks to meet the comprehensive biopsychosocial needs of its clients.

Lupus, however, is a complex illness, which is difficult to both diagnose and treat and much effort is required to locate and then assist those with the disease. A concerted coordinated approach, therefore, is appropriate in assisting those with lupus. While physicians are best suited to treat the physical manifestations of lupus, social workers in settings such as The S.L.E. Lupus Foundation are well-suited for addressing the biopsychosocial needs of lupus patients. Based on the apparent success of organizations such as the S.L.E. Lupus Foundation, future research should investigate the impact of community-based social work and social work education on those with lupus.

REFERENCES

Alarcón, G.S., McGwin Jr., G., Sanchez, M.L., Bastian, H.M., Fessler, B.J., Friedman, A.W., Baethge, B.A., . . . Reveille, J.D. (2004). Systemic lupus erythematosus in three ethnic groups. XIV. Poverty, wealth, and their influence on disease activity. *Arthritis Care & Research, 51*(1), 73–77.

Baker, K., & Pope, J. (2009). Employment and work disability in systemic lupus erythematosus: A systematic review. *Rheumatology, 48*(3), 281–284.

Beckerman, N.L., Auerbach, C., & Blanco, I. (2011). Psychosocial dimensions of SLE: Implications for the health care team. *Journal of Multidisciplinary Healthcare, 4*, 63–72.

Danoff-Burg, S., & Friedberg, F. (2009). Unmet needs of patients with systemic lupus erythematosus. *Behavioral Medicine, 35*(1), 5–13.

Donoghue, P.J., & Siegel, M.E. (2000). *Sick and tired of feeling sick and tired: Living with invisible chronic illness.* New York, NY: WW Norton & Company.

Fernández, M., Alarcón, G.S., Calvo-alén, J., Andrade, R., McGwin Jr, G., Vilá, L.M., & Reveille, J.D. (2007). A multiethnic, multicenter cohort of patients with systemic lupus erythematosus (SLE) as a model for the study of ethnic disparities in SLE. *Arthritis Care & Research, 57*(4), 576–584.

Greenhalgh, T. (2009). Patient and public involvement in chronic illness: Beyond the expert patient. *British Medical Journal, 338*(7695), 629–631.

Hardcastle, D.A., Powers, P.R., & Wenocur, S. (2011). *Community practice: Theories and skills for social workers.* New York, NY: Oxford University Press.

Hepworth, D.H., Rooney, R.H., Rooney, G.D., Strom-Gottfried, K., & Larsen, J.A. (2009). *Direct social work practice: Theory and skills.* Belmont, CA: Brooks/Cole Pub Co.

Jump, R.L., Robinson, M.E., Armstrong, A.E., Barnes, E.V., Kilbourn, K.M., & Richards, H.B. (2005). Fatigue in systemic lupus erythematosus: Contributions of disease activity, pain, depression, and perceived social support. *The Journal of Rheumatology, 32*(9), 1699–1705.

Kozora, E., Ellison, M., Waxmonsky, J., Wamboldt, F., & Patterson, T. (2005). Major life stress, coping styles, and social support in relation to psychological distress in patients with systemic lupus erythematosus. *Lupus, 14*(5), 363–372.

Moses, N., Wiggers, J., Nicholas, C., & Cockburn, J. (2005). Prevalence and correlates of perceived unmet needs of people with systemic lupus erythematosus. *Patient Education and Counseling, 57*(1), 30–38.

Pons-Estel, G.J., Alarcón, G.S., Scofield, L., Reinlib, L., & Cooper, G.S. (2010). Understanding the epidemiology and progression of systemic lupus erythematosus. *Seminars in Arthritis and Rheumatism, 39*(4), 257–268.

S.L.E. Lupus Foundation. (n.d.). About lupus. Retrieved from http://www.lupusny.org/about-lupus

Treharne, G.J., Kitas, G.D., Lyons, A.C., & Booth, D.A. (2005). Well-being in rheumatoid arthritis: The effects of disease duration and psychosocial factors. *Journal of Health Psychology, 10*(3), 457–474.

Wallace, D.J. (2008). *The lupus book: A guide for patients and their families.* New York, NY: Oxford University Press.

Whittemore, R., & Dixon, J. (2008). Chronic illness: The process of integration. *Journal of Clinical Nursing, 17*(7b), 177–187.

Yelin, E., Trupin, L., Katz, P., Criswell, L., Yazdany, J., Gillis, J., & Panopalis, P. (2007). Work dynamics among persons with systemic lupus erythematosus. *Arthritis Care & Research, 57*(1), 56–63.

Patients With Lupus: An Overview of Culturally Competent Practice

CARMEN ORTIZ HENDRICKS, DSW, ACSW

Wurzweiler School of Social Work, Yeshiva University,
New York, New York, USA

This article examines the need for culturally competent social work practice with systemic lupus erythematosus (SLE) patients. Because women are disproportionately impacted by this chronic autoimmune disease, and the majority of women are women of color, it is essential to address the related issues of health disparities among and between people of color, language and cultural barriers, and socioeconomic factors that impact those living with lupus. This article reviews the essential components of culturally competent social work practice, and provides implications for culturally competent program development, education and training, and direct service delivery.

INTRODUCTION

Systemic lupus erythematosus (SLE), a rheumatic autoimmune disease characterized by complex and changing disease manifestations, disproportionately affects women at a rate of 9:1 and certain racial/ethnic groups. SLE occurs more commonly in African-American and Afro-Caribbean females who are four times more likely to be diagnosed with SLE than their White, Caucasian counterparts. In fact, African-American females contract SLE at a younger age and the impact of the disease accrues more quickly (Alarcon et al., 1999; Alarcon et al, 2004; Cooper et al., 2002). There are numerous theories about the health disparities of SLE epidemiology (Urowitz et al., 2011) especially as it relates to disparities in incidence, prevalence, and long-term outcomes (Odutola & Ward, 2005). These findings suggest the importance of cultural competence when providing responsive and effective care to a vulnerable population. This article will highlight the research on health disparities among people of color with regards to SLE and the essential components of culturally competent social work practice when working with SLE patients. The implications for culturally competent program development, education and training will also be addressed.

LITERATURE REVIEW

Research on Health Disparities

As early as 1991, Petri and colleagues explored SLE disease manifestations along with racial and socioeconomic variables. They reported that African-American lupus patients generally had lower education, income and job status than Whites as well as less access to health care and poorer adherence to medical care (Petri, Perez-Gutthann, Longenacker, & Hochberg, 1991). Later research uncovered that African-American lupus patients have mortality rates at least three times as high as Whites (Alarcon, 2006; Bertoli, Vila, Reveille, & Alarcon, 2008; Cooper et al., 2002; Krishnan & Hubert, 2006; Reveille, Bartolucci, & Alarcon, 1990). SLE incidence, morbidity and mortality are all much higher among people of African descent than among Whites or other racial/ethnic groups in the United States (Bastian et al., 2002; Bastian et al., 2007; Odutola & Ward, 2005; Krishnan & Hubert, 2006). These findings are consistent with research on general health disparities in the United States where poverty and discrimination produce biased health outcomes for people of color (http://minorityhealth.hhs.gov/templates/browse. aspx?lvl=2&lvlID=54).

The LUMINA organization (LUpus in Minorities: NAture vs. nurture) has an ongoing SLE study since 1994 that has confirmed health disparities for patients of Hispanic and African-American ancestry (Alarcon et al., 1999, 2001, 2004, 2006; Chaiamnuay et al., 2007). In the LUMINA cohort, African Americans had more difficulty keeping follow-up medical appointments; Whites and Hispanics were the least likely to become lost to follow-up (Bertoli et al., 2006, 2007, 2008). Research also demonstrates that SLE patients who participate in Health Maintenance Organizations (HMOs) as opposed to private medical care were less likely to have outpatient surgery and hospital admissions (Yelin et al., 2007).

One striking study of the correlation of race and SLE found that "among 6521 hospitalized SLE patients in South Carolina, African Americans were more likely than Whites to experience both in-hospital mortality and mortality after one year following hospital discharge" (Anderson et. al., 2008,

p. 819). The researchers considered a range of socioeconomic variables and co-morbidity variables and came to the conclusion that African-American SLE patients had a 15% increased mortality risk compared to Whites (Anderson, Nietert, Kamen, & Gilkeson, 2008). Other studies argue that it is not race alone but poverty that explains the differential mortality rates among different racial/ethnic groups, and that race and class combined contributed to the health disparities across groups (Duran, Apte, & Alarcon, 2007; Fernandez et al., 2007; Hopkinson, Jenkinson, Muir, Doherty, & Powell, 2000; Lotstein et al., 1998; Walsh & Gilchrist, 2006). Throughout these studies, health disparities by age, race, and gender were prominent in the clinical and immunological features of recently diagnosed SLE patients (Kaslow & Masi, 1978; Lotstein et al., 1998; Cooper et al., 2002).

On October 31, 2011, the U.S. Department of Health and Human Services released a new survey to measure ethnicity, race, sex, disability status, and language preference to better track health disparity patterns and to aid in the development of health policies that are better suited to the nation's demographic diversity (USDHHS, 2011). HHS Secretary Kathleen Sebelius says of this initiative:

> It is our job to get a better understanding of why disparities occur and how to eliminate them. Improving the breadth and quality of our data collection and analysis on key areas, like race, ethnicity, sex, primary language and disability status, is critical to better understanding who we are serving. (USDHHS, 2011)

These efforts stem from the Patient Protection and Affordable Care Act, which mandated improved standards for the collection of health information. A standardized system for collecting health information should facilitate identifying the unique health challenges that often affect minority groups.

Research has thus far not shown why women are so prone to the manifestations of SLE or why women of color are so vulnerable to the disease. What is known is that SLE targets women over men 9:1 and people of color over Whites. All potential variables impacting SLE populations have been examined from age, race, gender, geographic location, nutrition, genetic makeup, and life style factors (Fernandez et al. 2007; Walsh & Gilchrist, 2006). Most likely it is a combination of these factors that contribute to these disparities and social workers should examine some of these key factors to enhance their culturally competent practice.

An Ecological Perspective

Historically, social workers are trained to utilize an ecological perspective (Germain, 1973), a dual concern for people and their environments, when assessing their work with individuals, families, groups and communities.

This perspective looks at the person-in-environment and includes among many variables biology and health, racial/ethnic identity, culture, gender and sexual orientation, social and familial situations, environmental factors, emotional and psychological functioning, spiritual and religious beliefs, and the financial and political structures that impact people's lives (Waters, Chang, Worsdall, & Ramsey-Goldman, 1996; Yazdany et al., 2007). Thus, a social worker looks at an SLE patient as a whole person connected to many aspects of their environment all of which are interacting with the illness. Utilizing a strengths perspective, the social worker looks for resiliency, capacity building, and sustainability within the patient's total environment that can effectively be used throughout the course of treatment (Saleebey, 2006). The social worker also looks for the patient's perceptions of health, mental health, and wellness rather than the medical model of symptoms and diagnosis. Above all, the social worker seeks to understand how different cultures perceive, identify, and respond to health care challenges such as SLE (Hendricks, 2003).

The social work approach is to provide psychosocial services to a person who has just learned that they have a potentially life-threatening illness by assessing and treating from a multimodal approach depending on the unique psychological and sociocultural context of each patient. A comprehensive and culturally competent social work approach with this population can include crisis intervention skills; assessing the severity of the patient's trauma and emotional reactions; providing psychoeducation to inform the patient about what is known about SLE; case management to enhance social support network; and group therapy to strengthen bonds among SLE patients that increase opportunities for emotional support and community building. This multimodal approach empowers those affected by the disease and enhances sustainability and promotes recovery. It helps patients understand what is happening to them; validates their experiences; normalizes what may feel like abnormal responses; prepares them to deal with the serious symptoms of SLE; and moves the recovery process forward.

Cultural Competence

Cultural competence is a set of congruent behaviors, attitudes, and policies that come together in a system or agency or among professionals and enable the system, agency, or professionals to work effectively in cross-cultural situations (NASW, 2000, p. 61). A cultural competence perspective (self-awareness, sensitivity, and competence) guides social workers in examining their practice especially as it relates to the workers' capacity to develop authentic relationships with persons who are culturally very similar or different. This includes the ability to understand the daily experience of people whose realities are different from the social worker's own; an appreciation of the social, political, organizational, and economic arrangements that maintain oppression, dominance, and privilege in society; and the physical, emotional, and psychological cost of dealing with stressful life situations. SLE patients reflect all these factors but especially the broader systemic factors that maintain health disparities in the United States.

Culturally competent social workers understand how the diagnosis of SLE is experienced differently by people based on their life experiences and their capacity to understand their status in society. For example, African-American women have a particular oppression and dominance history in the United States that informs their reaction to diagnosis, the health care system and treatment. Afro-Caribbeans reflect numerous cultures that all have their own unique set of beliefs and practices about health and illness, and Hispanic women, also from a myriad of origins, have numerous different ways of understanding health, illness, health care systems and treatments. Each of these unique cultures may present difficulty in accessing health care from culturally and linguistically competent health care professionals who do not understand their perceptions of health and well-being. Research shows that when there is concordance of race or ethnicity between patient and practitioner, patients are more likely to adhere to treatment and follow-up services (Gillis et al., 2007; Gonzalez, & Gonzalez-Ramos, 2005).

Fighting adversity with strength and resilience is built into the African-American and Hispanic woman's experience. Social workers need to help these women build on their resilience and determination to overcome all kinds of adversity from racism, sexism, and obstacles to health and well-being.

Furthermore, social workers will encounter SLE patients in a variety of agency settings from community based organizations, clinics, inpatient and outpatient facilities, and anywhere in the continuum of health care beginning with diagnosis, following treatment phases, and even through palliative care. Most social workers will not be familiar with SLE and the course of the disease. A commitment to continuing education in this area is strongly recommended for the ongoing development of cultural competence in social work practice and supervision in health care.

From an ecological perspective, the worker, with or without a full understanding of SLE, can see the person and the disease from an integrated perspective that both individualizes the person and their situation and appreciates the universal macro factors that impinge on the person's health and well-being. This includes an awareness of how human diversity affects life choices and adaptations. Race, class, gender, ethnicity, religious or spiritual beliefs, and sexual orientation limit or enhance life choices and one's ability to adapt to new and ever changing life events. Social workers need to keep these diversity factors in the forefront when dealing with SLE patients in order to understand their patients' situations and what issues may enhance their health and recovery.

This is more difficult than it appears. Social workers need to balance their own respective differences and similarities, the individual (micro) and the universal (macro), personal and professional values and beliefs about health and illness, and the private and the public face of SLE patients. "Attention only to similarities without attention to differences reinforces the orientation that all people are the same and invites ignoring or denial of difference. Attention only to difference without attention to similarities reinforces distancing, separation, and barriers between people" (Pinderhughes, 1989, p. 27). Each patient is a unique individual, but when a group of patients, for example women of color, is more affected by a particular problem, for example SLE, then the social worker needs to examine the reason why and address those factors as well.

Indicators for Cultural Competence

The National Association of Social Workers established *Standards for Cultural Competence in Social Work Practice* (2000) and more recently (2007) *Indicators for the Achievement of the NASW Standards for Cultural Competence in Social Work Practice.* The ten standards can be used to create goals and objectives for what constitutes cultural competence with lupus patients: (1) Professional Ethics & Values; (2) Self-Awareness; (3) Cross-Cultural Knowledge; (4) Cross-Cultural Skills; (5) Service Delivery; (6) Empowerment & Advocacy; (7) Diverse Workforce; (8) Professional Education; (9) Language Diversity; and (10) Cross-Cultural Leadership. Below are the indicators for Standard 4: Cross-Cultural Skills, all of which impact on work with SLE patients.

Three NASW indicators of cultural competence (#4, 6, & 11) are most relevant to social work practice with SLE patients who are of a different race/ethnicity/culture/class or gender.

STANDARD 4. CROSS-CULTURAL SKILLS

Social workers shall use appropriate methodological approaches, skills, and techniques that reflect the workers' understanding of the role of culture in the helping process.

Indicators

Culturally competent social workers will

1. Interact with persons from a wide range of cultures.
2. Display proficiency in discussing cultural difference with colleagues and clients.
3. ***Develop and implement a comprehensive assessment of clients in which culturally normative behavior is differentiated from problem or symptomatic behavior.***
4. Assess cultural strengths and limitations/challenges and their impact on individual and group functioning, and integrate this understanding into intervention plans.

5. *Select and develop appropriate methods, skills, and techniques that are attuned to their clients' cultural, multicultural, or marginal experiences in their environments.*
6. Adapt and use a variety of culturally proficient models.
7. Communicate effectively with culturally and linguistically different clients through language acquisition, proper use of interpreters, verbal and nonverbal skills, and culturally appropriate protocols.
8. Advocate for the use of interpreters who are both linguistically and culturally competent and prepared to work in the social services environment.
9. *Effectively employ the clients' natural support system in resolving problems, for example, folk healers, indigenous remedies, religious leaders, friends, family, and other community residents and organizations.*
10. Advocate, negotiate, and employ empowerment skills in their work with clients.
11. Consult with supervisors and colleagues for feedback and monitoring of performance and identify features of their own professional style that impede or enhance their culturally competent practice (NASW, 2000).

In short, this reflects the ecological model wherein the social worker helps the client adapt to his/her environment (health care), simultaneously facilitating a responsive adaptation from the environment to meet the clients' biopsychosocial needs. The social work practitioner should assess what cultural norms have been particularly useful in helping clients through difficult situations; recognizing that some cultures enjoy privilege while other cultures face oppression; and utilizing the client's natural support systems are extremely effective in dealing with women of color who are diagnosed with SLE.

In Standard 6: Empowerment and Advocacy, all indicators are concerned with changing the societal system to include health equity for all people in need of health services. Indicators 4, 6 and 9 target the systems and policies that impede health equity (NASW, 2007). SLE patients can become more cognizant of their own power in dealing with the health care system and their treatment plans. There are partner organizations like LUMINA that are working to understand the disease, its epidemiology and cure. By advocating for themselves, SLE patients are advocating for future lupus patients, their families and caregivers.

Standard 6. Empowerment and Advocacy

Social workers shall be aware of the effect of social policies and programs on diverse client populations, advocating for and with clients whenever appropriate.

Indicators

Culturally competent social workers will

1. Advocate for public policies that respect the cultural values, norms, and behaviors of diverse groups and communities.
2. Select appropriate intervention strategies to help colleagues, collaborating partners, and institutional representatives examine their own awareness and lack of awareness and behavioral consequences of the "isms," such as exclusionary behaviors, or oppressive policies by
   a. assessing level of readiness for feedback and intervention of the dominant group member.
   b. selecting either education, dialogue, increased intergroup contact, social advocacy, or social action as a strategy.
   c. participating in social advocacy and social action to better empower diverse clients and communities at the local, state, and/or national level.
3. *Use practice methods and approaches that help the client facilitate a connection with their own power in a manner that is appropriate for their cultural context.*
4. *Provide support to diverse cultural groups who are advocating on their own behalf.*
5. *Partner, collaborate, and ally with client groups in advocacy efforts.*
6. *Work to increase the client group's skills and sense of self-efficacy as social change agents.*
7. Demonstrate appropriate thoughtfulness regarding the role of their own personal values, particularly in terms of when to assert personal values during advocacy work and when to avoid imposing personal values during empowerment work.
8. Demonstrate intentional effort to assure that one does not impose one's own personal values in practice. (NASW, 2000)

This indicator emphasizes that social work practice with the lupus should be particularly aware of the potential vulnerability of disenfranchised women and endeavor to support client self-determination empowerment. The social worker must be vigilant about trying to understand how the client will perceive their illness and care through the lens of their own unique culture an subcultures.

STANDARD 9. LANGUAGE DIVERSITY

Health care organizations should maintain a current demographic, cultural, and epidemiological profile of the community as well as a needs assessment to accurately plan for and implement services that respond to the cultural and linguistic characteristics of the service area (USDHHS, 2011). The U.S. Department of Health and Human Services has established their own Standards for Culturally and Linguistically Appropriate Services (CLAS) and Standard 11 is of particular importance when working with SLE patients. Social workers should advocate including SLE as a significant health issue in minority communities, and requiring the Office of Minority Health to include an epidemiological profile of SLE at the federal level.

Regarding the seismic shifts in the cultural composition of U.S. residents, the 2010 U.S. Census shows the Hispanic population, the fastest growing racial/ethnic group in the United States, reaching 50.5 million or 16.3% of the U.S. population, there is indeed a need to recruit and retain more culturally and linguistically competent health care providers to serve the diverse patients in diverse communities (USDHHS, 2011). The U.S. Department of Health and Human Services Office of Minority Health cites language/cultural barriers, lack of access to preventive care, and the lack of health insurance as the primary barriers to Hispanic health (USDHHS, 2011).

CONCLUSION

Achieving cultural competence is an ongoing, lifelong process for all health care providers. "Cultural competence does not come naturally to any social worker and requires a high level of professionalism and sophistication, yet how culturally competent practitioners are trained is not clear in professional education or practice" (Hendricks, 2003, p. 75). As the profession begins to understand the components of culturally competent practice, it informs social work education and training on ways to better prepare practitioners, and vice versa. At one time, educators thought it was enough to help social work students develop cultural self-awareness and sensitivity to personal biases and stereotypes. The following recommendations would help address cultural competency practices with SLE patients:

1. Continued research into the epidemiology of SLE particularly as it affects women of color;
2. Further development of psychoeducational resources that decrease stigma and enhance competence for both patient and health care providers;
3. Involve SLE patients, especially women of color, in the development and implementation of trainings for health care providers;
4. Integrate culturally competent approaches in all aspects of diagnosis and treatment plans with SLE patients;
5. Advocate for the necessary resources to meet the needs of vulnerable women of color who are the majority of patients with SLE;
6. Recruit more culturally and linguistically competent health care providers.

Today, social workers and social work educators know that cultural competence implies more than just being aware of personal values, attitudes, and worldview perspectives. Cultural competence requires an understanding of within- and between-group differences; identity development; power, privilege, and oppression; and the experience of living with multiple identities and social statuses. The development of culturally competent knowledge, skills, and values is critical for social workers working with lupus patients today. Of particular importance is the changing population demographics (U.S. Census, 2010), data on the underutilization of health/mental health services by clients of color, and particularly Hispanics (Gonzalez & Gonzalez-Ramos, 2005), and the profession's ethical standards on diversity (NASW, 1999, ES 1.05).

REFERENCES

Alarcon, G.S., Bastian, H.M., Beasley, T.M., Roseman, J.M., Tan, F.K., Fessler, B.J., Vila, L.M., & McGwin, G. (2006). Systemic lupus erythematosus in a multi-ethnic cohort (LUMINA) XXXII: [corrected] contributions of admixture and socioeconomic status to renal involvement. *Lupus, 15*(1), 26–31.

Alarcon, G.S., Friedman, A.W., Straaton, K.V., Moulds, J.M., Lisse, J., Bastian, H.M., McGwin, G., Jr., Bartolucci, A.A., Roseman, J.M., & Reveille, J.D. (1999). Systemic lupus erythematosus in three ethnic groups: III. A comparison of characteristics early in the natural history of the LUMINA cohort. LUpus in MInority populations: NAture vs. Nurture. *Lupus, 8*(3), 197–209.

Alarcon, G.S., McGwin, G., Jr., Bastian, H.M., Roseman, J., Lisse, J., Fessler, B.J., Friedman, A.W., & Reveille, J.D. (2001). Systemic lupus erythematosus in three ethnic groups. VII [correction of VIII]. Predictors of early mortality in the LUMINA cohort. LUMINA Study Group. *Arthritis and Rheumatism, 45*(2), 191–202.

Alarcon, G.S., McGwin, G., Jr., Sanchez, M.L., Bastian, H.M., Fessler, B.J., Friedman, A.W., Baethge, B.A., Roseman, J., Reveille, & J.D. (2004). Systemic lupus erythematosus in three ethnic groups. XIV. Poverty, wealth, and their influence on disease activity. *Arthritis and Rheumatism, 51*(1), 73–77.

Anderson, E., Nietert, P.J., Kamen, D.L., & Gilkeson, G.S. (2008). Ethnic disparities among patients with systemic lupus erythematosus in South Carolina. *Journal of Rheumatology, 35*(5), 819–825.

Bastian, H.M., Alarcon, G.S., Roseman, J.M., McGwin, G., Jr., Vila, L.M., Fessler, B.J., & Reveille, J.D. (2007). Systemic lupus erythematosus in a multiethnic US cohort (LUMINA) XL II: factors predictive of new or worsening proteinuria. *Rheumatology, 46*(4), 683–689.

Bastian, H.M., Roseman, J.M., McGwin, G., Jr., Alarcon, G.S., Friedman, A.W., Fessler, B.J., Baethge, B.A., & Reveille, J.D. (2002). Systemic lupus erythematosus in three ethnic groups. XII. Risk factors for lupus nephritis after diagnosis. *Lupus, 11*(3), 152–160.

Bertoli, A.M., Fernandez, M., Alarcon, G.S., Vila, L.M., & Reveille, J.D. (2007). Systemic lupus erythematosus in a multiethnic US cohort LUMINA (XLI): Factors predictive of self-reported work disability. *Annals of the Rheumatic Diseases*, *66*(1), 12–17.

Bertoli, A.M., Fernandez, M., Calvo-Alen, J., Vila, L.M., Sanchez, M.L., Reveille, J.D., & Alarcon, G.S. (2006). Systemic lupus erythematosus in a multiethnic U.S. cohort (LUMINA) XXXI: Factors associated with patients being lost to follow-up. *Lupus*, *15*(1), 19–25.

Bertoli, A.M., Vila, L.M., Reveille, J.D., & Alarcon, G.S. (2008). Systemic lupus erythematosus in a multiethnic US cohort (LUMINA) LIII: Disease expression and outcome in acute onset lupus. *Annals of the Rheumatic Diseases*, *67*(4), 500–504.

Chaiamnuay, S., Bertoli, A.M., Roseman, J.M., McGwin, G., Apte, M., Duran, S., Vila, L.M., & Reveille, J.D., & Alarcon, G.S. (2007). African-American and Hispanic ethnicities, renal involvement and obesity predispose to hypertension in systemic lupus erythematosus: Results from LUMINA, a multiethnic cohort (LUMINAXLV). *Annals of the Rheumatic Diseases*, *66*(5), 618–622.

Cooper, G.S., Parks, C.G., Treadwell, E.L., St Clair, E.W., Gilkeson, G.S., Cohen, P.L., Roubey, R.A., & Dooley, M.A. (2002). Differences by race, sex and age in the clinical and immunologic features of recently diagnosed systemic lupus erythematosus patients in the southeastern United States. *Lupus*, *11*(3), 161–167.

Duran, S., Apte, M., & Alarcon, G.S. (2007). Poverty, not ethnicity, accounts for the differential mortality rates among lupus patients of various ethnic groups. *Journal of National Medical Association*, *99*(10), 1196–1198.

Fernandez, M., Alarcon, G.S., Calvo-Alen, J., Andrade, R., McGwin, G., Jr., Vila, L.M., & Reveille, J.D. (2007). A multiethnic, multicenter cohort of patients with systemic lupus erythematosus (SLE) as a model for the study of ethnic disparities in SLE. *Arthritis and Rheumatism*, *57*(4), 576–584.

Germain, C.B. (1973). An ecological perspective in casework. *Social Casework*, *54*(6), 323–330.

Gillis, J.Z., Yazdany, J., Trupin, L., Julian, L., Panopalis, P., Criswell, L.A., Katz, P., & Yelin, E. (2007). Medicaid and access to care among persons with SLE. *Arthritis and Rheumatism*, *57*(4), 601–607.

Gonzalez, M.J., & Gonzalez-Ramos, G. (2005). *Mental health care for new Hispanic immigrants: Innovative approaches in contemporary clinical practice*. New York, NY: Haworth Press.

Hendricks, C.O. (2003). Learning and teaching culturally competent social work practice. *Journal of Teaching in Social Work*, *23*(1/2), 73–86.

Hopkinson, N.D., Jenkinson, C., Muir, K.R., Doherty, M., & Powell, R.J. (2000). Racial group, socioeconomic status, and the development of persistent proteinuria in systemic lupus erythematosus. *Annals of the Rheumatic Diseases*, *59*(2), 116–119.

Kaslow, R.A., & Masi, A.T. (1978). Age, sex, and race effects on mortality from systemic lupus erythematosus in the United States. *Arthritis and Rheumatism*, *21*(4), 473–479.

Krishnan, E., & Hubert, H.B. (2006). Ethnicity and mortality from systemic lupus erythematosus in the US. *Annals of the Rheumatic Diseases*, *65*(11), 1500–1505.

Lotstein, D.S., Ward, M.M., Bush, T.M., Lambert, R.E., van Vollenhoven, R., & Neuwelt, C.M. (1998). Socioeconomic status and health in women with systemic lupus erythematosus. *Journal of Rheumatology*, *25*(9), 1720–1729.

National Association of Social Workers. (1999). *Code of ethics of the national association of social workers*. Washington, DC: NASW Press.

National Association of Social Workers. (2000). Cultural competence in the social work profession. In *Social work speaks: NASW policy statements* (5th ed.). Washington, DC: NASW Press.

National Association of Social Workers. (2007). *Indicators for the achievement of the NASW standards for cultural competence in social work practice*. Washington, DC: NASW Press.

Odutola, J.M., & Ward, H. (2005). Ethnic and socioeconomic disparities in health among patients with rheumatic disease. *Current Opinions in Rheumatology*, 7(2), 147–152.

Petri, M., Perez-Gutthann, S., Longenecker, J.C., & Hochberg, M. (1991). Morbidity of systemic lupus erythematosus: role of race and socioeconomic status. *American Journal of Medicine*, 91(4), 345–353.

Pinderhughes, E. (1989). *Understanding race, ethnicity and power: The key to efficacy in clinical practice*. New York, NY: The Free Press.

Reveille, J.D., Bartolucci, A., & Alarcon, G.S. (1990). Prognosis in systemic lupus erythematosus. Negative impact of increasing age at onset, black race, and thrombocytopenia, as well as causes of death. *Arthritis and Rheumatism*, 33(1), 37–48.

Saleebey, D. (2006). *The strengths perspective in social work practice*. New York, NY: Allyn & Bacon.

Urowitz, M., Gladman, D., Ibanez, D., Fortin, P., Bae, S., Gordon, C., . . . Aranow, C. (2011). Evolution of disease burden over 5 years in a multicentre inception SLE cohort. *Arthritis Care and Research (Hoboken)*.

U.S. Census (2010). Census Bureau Homepage www.census.gov

U.S. Department of Health and Human Services Office of Minority Health. (2011). Retrieved from http://minorityhealth.hhs.gov/templates/browse.aspx?lvl=2&lvlID=54

Walsh, S.J., & Gilchrist, A. (2006). Geographical clustering of mortality from systemic lupus erythematosus in the United States: Contributions of poverty, Hispanic ethnicity and solar radiation. *Lupus*, 15(10), 662–670.

Waters, T.M., Chang, R.W., Worsdall, E., & Ramsey-Goldman, R. (1996). Ethnicity and access to care in SLE. *Arthritis Care Research*, 9(6), 492–500.

Yazdany, J., Gillis, J.Z., Trupin, L., Katz, P., Panopalis, P., Criswell, L.A., & Yelin, E. (2007). Association of socioeconomic and demographic factors with utilization of rheumatology subspecialty care in systemic lupus erythematosus. *Arthritis and Rheumatism*, 57(4), 593–600.

Yelin, E., Trupin, L., Katz, P., Criswell, L.A., Yazdany, J., Gillis, J., & Panopalis, P. (2007). Impact of health maintenance organizations and fee-for-service on health care utilization among people with systemic lupus erythematosus. *Arthritis and Rheumatism*, 57(3), 508–515.

Research Studies and Their Implications for Social Work Practice in a Multidisciplinary Center for Lupus Care

SU JIN KIM, LCSW

*Department of Social Work Programs, Hospital for
Special Surgery, New York, New York, USA*

PRETIMA PERSAD, MPH, DORUK ERKAN, MD,
and KYRIAKOS KIROU, MD

*Division of Rheumatology, Hospital for Special Surgery,
New York, New York, USA*

ROBERTA HORTON, LCSW, ACSW

*Department of Social Work Programs, Hospital for
Special Surgery, New York, New York, USA*

JANE E. SALMON, MD

*Division of Rheumatology, Hospital for Special Surgery,
New York, New York, USA*

*The complexity of systemic lupus erythematosus (SLE) and its
psychosocial impact creates management challenges that require
a multidisciplinary team approach for optimal patient care
and outcomes. This article provides a brief report on current
lupus-related research studies at the Mary Kirkland Center for
Lupus Care at Hospital for Special Surgery. Studies and their
social work implications highlight a comprehensive, integrated
model for research, education, and patient care emphasizing*

The Mary Kirkland Center for Lupus Care is funded, in part, by the Mary Kirkland
Center for Lupus Research through support from Rheuminations, Inc. The authors thank
Glendalee Ramon (Hospital for Special Surgery Research Assistant) for her contributions in
the preparation of this article.

interdisciplinary collaboration. Both basic science and clinical research are discussed, with a focus on the role of social workers as an integral part of the health care team in providing assessments and interventions and as support for patients in research studies.

INTRODUCTION

The complexity of systemic lupus erythematosus (SLE) and its psychosocial impact creates management challenges that require a multidisciplinary approach to better ensure optimal patient outcomes. Additionally, the increased interest in lupus research has generated the need to more efficiently recruit for studies.

In 2009, Hospital for Special Surgery (HSS) established the SLE-Antiphospholipid Syndrome (APS) Center of Excellence and The Mary Kirkland Center for Lupus Care (MKCLC) with the primary goal of integrating patient care, patient and physician education, and clinical and psychosocial research (Persad et al., 2010). Key staff play a pivotal role in implementing this collaborative model. The Center Manager coordinates and matches patients to appropriate studies that patients may be eligible for by collaborating closely with the Center's Research Coordinators. Additional important support roles include the Center's Nurse Practitioner, who performs initial patient assessments of preventative health measures and the Center's social workers, who provide psychosocial assessments and screen for high risk needs needs (Persad et al., 2010). MKCLC provides patient education about SLE; depression screenings; cardiovascular disease (CVD) prevention counseling; social work assessments and referrals; and opportunities to learn about and participate in clinical and observational research in SLE. In close collaboration with MKCLC, HSS' Department of Social Work Programs offers more free, social work–led support and education programs for people with lupus and their families than any other hospital in the nation: LANtern® (Lupus Asian Network); SLE Workshop, LupusLine®; Charla de Lupus (Lupus Chat)®; VOICES 60+. The purpose of this article is to describe the MKCLC's current and ongoing research studies and their implications for social work education and practice.

THE SLE AND APS REGISTRY AND REPOSITORY: A PATHWAY TO RESEARCH

As the "backbone" of research, clinical disease registries help to inform research opportunities. As an established medical database in the

Rheumatology Division at HSS, the Registry and Repository support and promote basic science and clinical research into the mechanisms of disease susceptibility and pathways that cause autoimmunity and organ damage. Better understanding of disease etiology will allow for the development of more effective therapeutic agents. The Registry and Repository contain longitudinal clinical data, demographic information, and biological specimens. Data are updated and samples are collected at the time patients visit their physicians. This collection, containing over 1,100 SLE patients, is a resource for identifying patients for clinical studies and translational studies at HSS and with other institutions. The Registry and its activities enable patients to be a part of a community that is mutually committed to understanding the basis of their disease and finding treatments. It guides patients to feel supported in their medical care, but also helps to bridge patients to resources for their psychosocial needs through referrals by the Registry study coordinators.

Parallel to this is the opportunity for social workers to enhance their clinical practice and attention to the biopsychosocial factors impacting patients' lives, through their familiarity with this research. For example, Lupus Center medical conferences held weekly bring together physicians of multiple specialties, nurses, researchers, research assistants/coordinators, and social workers. These conferences are an excellent venue for teaching "case to cause" in social work education. Patient cases are discussed where both medical and psychosocial factors are reviewed, integrating the most current lupus-related research. Both new and experienced social workers have an opportunity to connect their clinical work to both patient care and research. While there are numerous clinical and psychosocial studies at any given time, those that have particular relevance for social workers in health care are highlighted below.

PREDICTORS OF PREGNANCY OUTCOME: BIOMARKERS IN ANTIPHOSPHOLIPID ANTIBODY SYNDROME AND SYSTEMIC LUPUS ERYTHEMATOSUS—PROMISSE

The PROMISSE Study, supported by the National Institute of Arthritis, Musculoskeletal and Skin Diseases, seeks to identify markers that are predictive of serious pregnancy complications in patients who have lupus. It is an ongoing, multicenter, prospective observational study of 700 pregnant patients, grouped and analyzed according to the presence or absence of antiphospholipid antibodies and preexisting SLE. Antiphospholipid antibodies (aPL) are abnormal circulating proteins associated with blood clots and pregnancy complications, and they are important to note since approximately 30% of patients with lupus also have aPL. We obtain and analyze detailed medical and obstetrical information during the course of pregnancy and serial blood specimens for markers of inflammation and placental growth factors. DNA and RNA are studied to identify inherited factors and to characterize the patterns of genes that are activated during the course of complicated and uncomplicated pregnancies, respectively. Characterization of clinically applicable markers that predict poor pregnancy outcomes should provide the necessary groundwork for interventional trials in patients at risk for fetal loss, and may eventually result in a means of preventing pregnancy complications, including miscarriage, preterm birth, fetal growth restriction, and preeclampsia (characterized by hypertension, protein in the urine, and placental insufficiency) in lupus patients. An important component of support to the patients is the role of research coordinators, who not only meet monthly with them, but regularly attend obstetric appointments with patients, developing a partnership of advocacy and support.

A lupus patient's pregnancy can be filled with much joy, but also worry and concern in light of risk factors and the potential likelihood of complications during pregnancy. Knowledge of a 23% rate of miscarriages during pregnancy for SLE patients (Smyth et al., 2010) can exacerbate these concerns. In practice, social workers collaborating closely with research coordinators, often serve as a "touch point," to explore these concerns in greater depth, and to refer patients for peer support to other lupus patients who have gone through similar experiences. At times, high-risk pregnancies can pose ethical dilemmas for health care staff when pregnant women have challenging complications. The beliefs, values, attitudes, and judgments of a health care team can sometimes be in conflict with a patient, spouse and family's strong desire to have a child. For example, a patient with a strong spiritual or religious belief, experiencing a high risk pregnancy, may choose to "leave it in God's hands." In these situations, in order to better support the patient's wishes, social workers can help to facilitate and advocate for them during their pregnancy by mediating difficult conversations between medical staff and patients and their families, such as when termination of a pregnancy is being considered, or when there are a number of high-risk factors that may potentially harm the pregnant patient. In some cases, social workers can also intervene by calling for a Medical Ethics Meeting to review a patient's situation with the patient, family, and health care team in order to further clarify those risks and to make sure that the patient's safety is not at serious risk and that the patient's wishes are being carried out. Additionally, social workers are readily available when a patient has had a pregnancy loss to provide grief counseling and resources. This collaboration between patients, physicians, research coordinators, and social workers becomes an enormous support for lupus patients during this significant life event.

The unique partnership between social workers and research coordinators also provides opportunities for education of social work staff and interns. At bimonthly social work journal clubs, peer-reviewed articles are reviewed and discussed as a group. One such meeting, held with a focus on research initiatives, was facilitated by a social worker from our research division. This forum brought together social workers from both sides of the field to explore clinical interventions, research, and ethical issues.

COGNITION AND SLE STUDIES

Cognitive dysfunction is a clinical condition that results from abnormalities in certain areas of the brain related to attention/working memory, executive function, verbal/visual learning, memory, visual spatial functions, and motor skills. It may occur in almost half of SLE patients, and at some time in their disease, memory and executive functions may be particularly vulnerable (Erkan, Kozora, & Lockshin, 2011). Cognitive dysfunction is a manifestation of central nervous system involvement of SLE.

Studies analyzing cognition in lupus patients aim to provide information regarding the prevalence and mechanism of cognitive dysfunction. One such pilot study entails the administration of a neuropsychiatric battery of paper and pencil tests followed by a neuroimaging session designed to capture brain activity at rest as well as while performing specific simple tasks. The study compares SLE patients without aPL (antiphospholipid antibodies) positivity and without neuropsychiatric syndromes (as both also can be related to cognitive dysfunction) with aPL-positive non-SLE patients; and it correlates neuroimaging (functional MRI and diffusion tensor imaging) to cognitive function in these two patient groups simultaneously (Erkan et al., 2011).

It is important to note that cognitive dysfunction can significantly impair quality of life. A better understanding of the nature and pathogenesis of cognitive dysfunction in SLE is therefore critical to developing rational management approaches in these populations. These ongoing studies looking at cognition serve to normalize lupus patients' self reports of forgetfulness, memory loss, and often reports of "brain fog" that can cause emotional distress and isolation. For example, patients who are high functioning nevertheless can experience "brain fog" leading to difficulties with memory (i.e., forgetting where you placed your keys, forgetting your appointments, etc.). In practice, social workers can open up a dialogue with patients around how these cognitive changes impact self-esteem, self-efficacy, as well as individual and family roles and lifestyle changes. Identifying practical coping methods and recruiting help and support through family members and loved ones, social work practitioners can assist patients with adaptation. In consultation with the health care team, cognitive rehabilitation strategies and neuropsychiatric consultations can be explored for better management.

ASSESSING FACTORS THAT INFLUENCE APPOINTMENT COMPLIANCE RATES: A PILOT STUDY

A recent study by Osterberg and Blaschke (2005) suggests that missed patient appointments can interfere with treatment adherence and lead to poor health outcomes. The primary objective of this two-phase standard-of-care study was to analyze the demographic and clinical characteristics of a select cohort of lupus patients in the MKCLC clinic who missed appointments over one year compared to those who did not. The secondary objective was to determine the effectiveness of a "telephone intervention" on appointment compliance. Surprisingly, there were no significant changes in appointment compliance after the introduction of the telephone intervention. The study showed that poor appointment compliance is more likely related to socioeconomic factors than to demographics, lupus manifestations, or confirmation of appointments. Preliminary data suggested that improving transportation services and providing access to temporary childcare for medical appointments may aide in increasing appointment compliance rates in a clinic setting (Persad, Kim, Kirou, & Erkan, 2011).

These preliminary findings have several implications for social work practice. Often, there can be an assumption by health care staff that patients' poor compliance with their appointments or treatment is due to forgetfulness or lack of engagement. This pilot study validates that patients do in fact have external barriers that can sometimes get in the way of seeking treatment. Its findings highlight the importance of our social work role in exploring with patients psychosocial and environmental circumstances that may interfere with their lupus treatment. More tailored interventions by social workers and the health care team that addresses patients' specific barriers may be helpful in solving concrete barriers such as transportation, child care, and job scheduling concerns. Although changing systems at a large clinic/practice may be challenging, thinking "outside the box" in finding solutions for individual patient barriers may, in the long run, help to increase patient adherence and ultimately, have patients know that the team cares and is committed to finding positive solutions for patients.

CARDIOVASCULAR DISEASE (CVD) AND SLE: A STUDY OF A PATIENT COUNSELING PROGRAM

SLE patients are at increased risk for atherosclerotic cardiovascular disease (myocardial infarction and strokes). Accelerated atherosclerosis, a premature hardening of the arteries, is related to lupus itself, as well as traditional CVD risk factors (e.g., hypertension, elevated cholesterol, smoking). In addition, patients with or without SLE, who have aPL, are at increased risk for blood clots in arteries and veins. A study to determine the satisfaction of

SLE and/or aPL-positive patients who participate in a counseling program has been developed to increase the awareness of CVD risk factors as well as thrombosis prevention strategies. This free-of-charge counseling program, partially supported by the New York Community Trust, provides a basic assessment of and education about CVD and thrombosis risk factors in SLE and/or aPL-positive patients. At the end of the counseling, patients receive tailored lifestyle recommendations, referrals to nutrition and physical therapy departments (as needed), and they also complete an anonymous survey to evaluate the program (Haiduc et al., 2009). This evolving 3-year longitudinal analysis of patients in the counseling program will determine whether the program is effective in decreasing the prevalence of cardiovascular disease risk factors.

The CVD counseling program models a more integrated, preventative care system where the health care team collaborates together for patient care, support, and education. It emphasizes a team approach of exploring patients' lifestyle and psychosocial barriers to provide patients with continued, ongoing support for better outcomes. Like lupus, CVD factors may be largely invisible. Patients may be finding out for the first time about their CVD risks, bringing about increased anxiety and overwhelming feelings of having to cope with more than one illness. Studies have shown that CVD is a longitudinal risk factor of depression in SLE patients (Julian et al., 2011) emphasizing the interplay between health and mental health conditions. For social work education, as a new social worker and intern, this program models well how public health issues can be addressed utilizing collaborative, interdisciplinary interventions that takes into account the "whole" patient. Patients report feeling burdened with multiple, complex diagnoses that are hard to manage, in addition to their other psychosocial needs. Social workers play an integral role in working with the patient and team to optimize opportunities for success in patients meeting their health goals. Self-care, improved nutrition, exercise, coming in for regularly scheduled medical appointments, and follow-up require a certain amount of patient activation. Social workers can effectively intervene to evaluate, support, and encourage patients' participation in these specific areas.

UTILIZING A DEPRESSION-SCREENING TOOL: A STUDY TO IDENTIFY DEPRESSION IN LUPUS PATIENTS

Studies have demonstrated that patients with SLE exhibit high levels of depression, which can adversely affect adherence to medical treatment and health outcomes (Julian et al., 2009). As part of our overall routine care at MKCLC, patients are evaluated by our social workers who assess medical and psychiatric history, coping and adaptation to their lupus, social supports and family systems, and non-medical needs such as assistance with homecare and transportation services. The MKCLC has been recently utilizing the Patient Health Questionnaire (PHQ9) depression screening tool, which is validated (Martin, Rief, Klaiberg, & Braehler, 2006) and has a record of effectiveness in primary care clinics (Kroneke, Spitzer, & Williams, 2001).

A study is underway analyzing rates of depression at MKCLC and looking at whether patients seek out mental health treatment when referred. The study results may provide answers to whether with mental health referrals and with treatment, patients report better coping and satisfaction in their overall medical care. Based on the preliminary analysis, we have learned that by incorporating a brief screening tool during a routine psychosocial evaluation, we can better identify depression and its severity, and we can facilitate a discussion around a patient's adaptation and coping (Kim et al., 2011). It creates an opportunity for the social worker to provide psychoeducation on depression and mental health referrals as part of overall lupus medical care during a routine appointment. Integrating social work assessments with an eye toward mental health, specifically depression, as part of the overall standard of care for all lupus patients, helps to see the lupus patient as a whole person and counteracts the tendency to segregate medical treatment from mental health treatment. The results of the PHQ9 can serve as a tool for assessing a patient's coping and strengths as well as for intervening with motivational and response prevention techniques to further help target one's psychosocial interventions. This ongoing social work study is an example highlighting how routine social work intervention and practices can lead to exploring social work opportunities that model evidence-based practice and how ultimately, this may lead to improvement in our patients' quality of life.

CONCLUSION

As part of a comprehensive model of care, the ongoing research studies conducted at MKCLC provide substantive opportunities for social work to integrate professional practice, and social work knowledge to optimize patient care and outcomes. We have provided examples of how patients who participate as research subjects, and the research environment itself, creates a powerful context for social work assessment and intervention regarding the psychosocial impact of these lupus-related realities.

In addition, such an environment can serve as a fertile training ground for both social work interns and social workers who are new to the field to learn the state of the art from case conferences, medical grand rounds, and other forums where we engage the entire health care team to create and implement plans to enhance the quality of life for patients with lupus. Social workers are a core element of this process and of the community of providers, and they empower and activate patients' further engagement in their own health management.

REFERENCES

Erkan, D., Kozora, E., & Lockshin, M.D. (2011). Cognitive dysfunction and white matter abnormalities in antiphospholipid syndrome. *Pathophysiology, 18*(1), 93–102.

Haiduc, I., Richey, M., Tzakas, S., Konstantellis, L., Pollino-Tanner, J., & Erkan, D. (2009). Cardiovascular disease prevention counseling program for Systemic Lupus Erythematosus and antiphosholipid antibody (aPL) positive patients. *Arthritis & Rheumatism, 60*(10), S479–480.

Julian, L.J., Tonner, C., Yelin, E., Yazdany, J., Trupin, L., Criswell, L.A., & Katz, P.P. (2011). Cardiovascular and disease-related predictors of depression in systemic lupus erythematosus. *Arthritis Care & Research, 63*(4), 542–549.

Julian, L.J., Yelin, E., Yazdany, J., Panopalis, P., Trupin, L., Criswell, L.A., & Katz, P. (2009). Depression, medication adherence, and service utilization in systemic lupus Erythematosus. *Arthritis & Rheumatism, 61*(2), 240–246.

Kim, S.J., Persad, P., Richey, M., Seehaus, M., Horton, R., Kirou, K., Erkan, D., & Barnhill, J. (2011). Piloting a Patient Health Questionnaire Depression Screening Tool in a hospital-based multi-disciplinary lupus clinic. *Arthritis & Rheumatism Abstract Supplement*, 2411, S938.

Kroneke, K., Spitzer, R.L., & Williams, J.B. (2001). The PHQ-9: Validity of a brief depression severity measure. *Journal of General Internal Medicine, 16*(9), 606–613.

Martin, A., Rief, W., Klaiberg, A., & Braehler, E. (2006). Validity of the Brief Patient health Questionnaire Mood Scale (PHQ-9) in the general population. *General Hospital Psychiatry, 28*(1), 71–77.

Osterberg, L., & Blaschke, T. (2005). Adherence to medication. *New England Journal of Medicine, 353*, 487–497.

Persad, P., Kim, S.J., Kirou, K., & Erkan, D. (2011). Factors that influence appointment compliance rates in a multi-disciplinary specialized lupus clinic. *Arthritis & Rheumatism Abstract Supplement*, 867, S341.

Persad, P., Kim, S., Richey, M., Salmon, J., Erkan, D., & Kirou, K. (2010). The Mary Kirkland Center for Lupus Care (MKCLC): A multi-disciplinary specialized disease center. *Arthritis & Rheumatism, 62*(10), 58–68.

Smyth, A., Oliveira, G.H., Lahr, B.C., Bailey, K.R., Norby, S.M., & Garovic, V.D. (2010). A systematic review and meta-analysis of pregnancy outcomes in patients with systemic lupus erythematosus and lupus nephritis. *Clinical Journal of the American Society of Nephrology, 11*, 2060–2068.

INDEX

Note: Page numbers in **bold** type refer to figures
Page numbers in *italic* type refer to tables

INDEX

diet: anti-inflammatory 26–7; Standard American (SAD) 26
disability: work 15–16, 53, 65
discoid rash 2
disease: brain 4; cardiovascular 94–5; course *see* flares; kidney 3
disease activity: and illness perceptions 49–62; and locus of control 52, 56–8
Dixon, J.: and Whittemore, R. 64

ecological perspective: social work 79–80
Einstein Lupus Cohort (ELC): Bronx 17–20
emotional challenges: patients and families 33–48
empowerment and advocacy 83–4
epidemiology 2, 14
exercise and movement: Integrative Medicine 28

family: and psychosocial impact 37–8, 39, *see also* patients and families
flares 37, 38, 41–2, 44; disease course 5–6; mild 5; severe 5
Friedberg, F.: and Danoff-Burg, S. 35
Functional Medicine 23–4, 25

genetics 6–9
Get Into The Loop Hospital Tour 71
Goodman, D.: *et al* 51
governmental community social work 69
Gross, D.: Rowshandel, J. and Schudrich, W. 63–75

health: care providers 73; disparities research 78–9
Health Maintenance Organizations (HMOs) 78
Health Related Quality of Life (HRQoL) 16
Hebra, F. von 6
Hendricks, C.O. 77–88
Hispanics 14–15, 16, 53, 78, 81, 85, 86
Hospital for Special Surgery (HSS): Mary Kirkland Center for Lupus Care 89–97

illness: chronic and biopsychosocial needs 64
illness perceptions/beliefs: and disease activity 49–62; Multidimensional Health Locus of Control Scale (MHLOC) 52, 56–8; survey demographics 54; survey instrument 52–3; survey participants 52; survey sample characteristics 53–4; Systemic Lupus Erythematosus Questionnaire (SLENQ) 52, 54–5
immunology 6–9
immunosuppressants 5, 8
Institute for Functional Medicine (IFM) 23–4
Integrative Medicine: acupuncture 28, 30; autoimmune assessment and treatment 23–32; definition 23; exercise and movement 28; systemic lupus erythematosus (SLE) 25–31; treatment 26–8

Kamhi, E.: *et al* 17
Karlson, E.: *et al* 45
kidney disease 3
Kim, S.J.: *et al* 89–97
Kulczycka, L.: *et al* 35

laboratory criteria 4–5
language diversity 84–5
Lindner, H.: and Lederman, L. 35
Living Life Healthy with Lupus program (SLE Foundation) 71
locus of control: and disease activity 52, 56–8, 57
Long Island University (LIU): Department of Occupational Therapy 71–2
loss 42–3
low blood cell counts 4
LUMINA cohort 18, 78, 83
Lupus Agencies of New York State (LANYS) 69
Lupus Aquatics Program 72
Lupus Awareness Month: New York 69
Lupus Cooperative of New York (LCNY) 68
Lupus Research Institute (LRI) National Coalition 69

McElhone, K.: *et al* 51
marital strain 35
Mary Kirkland Center for Lupus Care (HSS): appointment compliance factors 94; cardiovascular disease 94–5; cognitive studies 93; depression 95–6; PROMISSE study 91–3; Registry and Repository 90–1; research 89–97
media: new 70–1
Medicaid 18, 38, 53
medical overview 1–11
Medical Symptoms/Toxicity Questionnaire (MSQ) 30
minority lupus patients 65
morbidity 14–15
mortality 6
Moses, N.: *et al* 34, 52, 54–5, 65
movement: and exercise 28
Multidimensional Health Locus of Control Scale (MHLOC) 52; multinomial analysis 56–8
mycophenolate mofetil 29

nasal ulcers 3
National Association of Social Workers (NASW) 82
Navarette-Navarette, N.: *et al* 59
needs: biopsychosocial 64; client biophysical 67; psychosocial 54–5; Systemic Lupus Erythematosus Needs Questionnaire (SLENQ) 34, 52, 54–5
networking: social 71
nutrition workshop 72

99

Social Work in Health Care

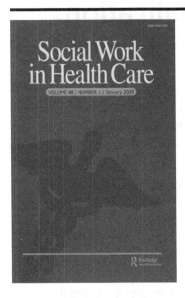

EDITOR: Gary Rosenberg, PhD
The Mount Sinai School of Medicine

ASSOCIATE EDITOR: Goldie Kadushin, PhD
University of Wisconsin-Milwaukee

MANAGING EDITOR: Andrew Weissman, PhD
The Mount Sinai School of Medicine
Email: andrew.weissman@mssm.edu

Visit the journal's web page at:
www.tandfonline.com/WSHC

Volume 52, 2013, 10 issues per year
Print ISSN: 0098-1389
Online ISSN 1541-034X

Social Work in Health Care remains one of the premier journals in the field that addresses both social work and health care issues. The journal presents vital peer-reviewed information on social work theory, practice, and administration as related to a variety of health care settings

Social Work in Health Care is edited by Gary Rosenberg, PhD, one of the most respected leaders in health social work. This outstanding journal publishes ten issues per year and brings readers the most important articles on research, leadership, clinical practice, management, education, collaborative relationships, social health policy, and ethical issues. The journal's special issues comprehensively discuss a single pertinent health care theme.

Readership: *Social Work in Health Care* presents practical and useful information for practitioners, administrators, educators, researchers, students, and professionals working at the crossroads of social work and health care.

In the US Contact:
Taylor & Francis - Customer Service Department
325 Chestnut Street, Philadelphia, PA 19106
Call Toll Free: 1-800-354-1420, press "4"
Fax: (215) 625-8914
Email: customerservice@taylorandfrancis.com

Outside the US Contact:
Informa UK Ltd - Customer Service
Sheepen Place, Colchester, Essex, CO3 3LP, UK
Tel: +44 (0)20 7017 5544,
Fax: +44 (0)20 7017 5198
Email: tf.enquiries@tfinforma.com

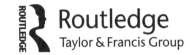

Routledge
Taylor & Francis Group

Journal of Social Work in Disability & Rehabilitation

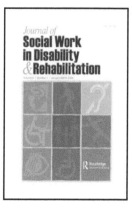

Editor:
Francis K. O. Yuen, DSW, ACSW
Professor, Division of Social Work
California State University - Sacramento,
6000 J Street, Sacramento, CA 95819
Email: fyuen@csus.edu

Visit the journal's web page at:
www.tandfonline.com/WSWD

Volume 11, 2012, 4 issues per year
Print ISSN: 1536-710X
Online ISSN: 1536-7118

The *Journal of Social Work in Disability & Rehabilitation* presents and explores issues related to disabilities and social policy, practice, research, and theory.

Reflecting the broad scope of social work in disability practice, this interdisciplinary journal examines vital aspects of the field - from innovative practice methods, legal issues, and literature reviews - to program descriptions and cutting-edge practice research. Use it to enhance your knowledge and skills and to broaden your professional understanding of the impact of the individual, family, group, community, and social services delivery system on persons with disabilities and on the rehabilitation process.

The *Journal of Social Work in Disability & Rehabilitation* is based on the concept that a disability can be understood through a number of perspectives, such as moral, medical, minority and social models. These models have influenced the education of social work students and the strategies used by professionals working with persons with disabilities. The journal provides new insight and understanding for students, educators, administrators, and professionals providing services to the community.

In the US Contact:
Taylor & Francis - Customer Service Dep artment
325 Chestnut Street, Philadelphia, PA 19106
Call Toll Free: 1-800-354-1420, press "4"
Fax: (215) 625-8914
Email: customerservice@taylorandfrancis.com

Outside the US Contact:
Informa UK Ltd - Customer Service
Sheepen Place, Colchester, Essex, CO3 3LP, UK
Tel: +44 (0)20 7017 5544,
Fax: +44 (0)20 7017 5198
Email: tf.enquiries@tfinforma.com

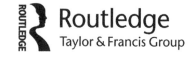

Journal of Family Social Work

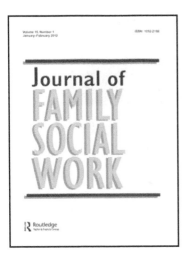

EDITOR
Pat Conway, PhD, LCSW
Senior Research Scientist
Essentia Institute of Rural Health
Maildrop: 5AV-2, 502 East Second Street
Duluth, MN 55805
Jfamilysocialwork@gmail.com

Visit the journal's web page at:
www.tandfonline.com/WFSW

Volume 15, 2012, 5 issues per year
Print ISSN: 1052-2158
Online ISSN: 1540-4072

In celebrating social workers' tradition of working with couples and families in their life context, the *Journal of Family Social Work* features articles which advance the capacity of practitioners to integrate research, theory building, and practice wisdom into their services to families. It is a journal of policy, clinical practice, and research directed to the needs of social workers working with couples and families.

The *Journal of Family Social Work* makes a unique attempt at balancing clinical relevance and academic exactitude. By uniting clinicians and researchers from social work, family enrichment, family therapy, family studies, family psychology and sociology, health and mental health, and child welfare, the journal stresses a blending of sociocultural contexts, the uniqueness of the family, and the person of the clinician. As an interdisciplinary forum, it provides a creative mixing of clinical innovation, practice wisdom, theory, and academic excellence.

In the US Contact:
Taylor & Francis - Customer Service Department
325 Chestnut Street, Philadelphia, PA 19106
Call Toll Free: 1-800-354-1420, press "4"
Fax: (215) 625-8914
Email: customerservice@taylorandfrancis.com

Outside the US Contact:
Informa UK Ltd - Customer Service
Sheepen Place, Colchester, Essex, CO3 3LP, UK
Tel: +44 (0)20 7017 5544,
Fax: +44 (0)20 7017 5198
Email: tf.enquiries@tfinforma.com

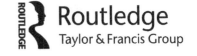

Routledge
Taylor & Francis Group

ROUTLEDGE

www.routledge.com/9780789037091

Related titles from Routledge

Social Work and Global Mental Health

Research and Practice Perspectives

Edited by Serge Dumont and Myreille St-Onge

This book presents respected experts, researchers, and clinicians providing the latest developments in social work knowledge and research. It discusses the latest in mental health research, information on violence, trauma and resilience, and social policies. Different mental health and social work approaches from around the world are examined in detail, including holistic, ethnopsychiatric, and interventions that place emphasis on recovery, empowerment, and social inclusion. This superb selection of presentations taken from the 4th International Conference on Social Work in Health and Mental Health held in Quebec, Canada in 2004 comprehensively examines the theme of how social work can contribute to the development of a world that values compassion and solidarity.

This book was originally published as a special issue of *Social Work in Mental Health*.

March 2009: 246 x 174: 306pp
Hb: 978-0-7890-3709-1
Pb: 978-0-7890-3710-7
Hb: £75 / $125 Pb: £25.99 / $49.95

For more information and to order a copy visit
www.routledge.com/9780789037091

Available from all good bookshops